ANAESTHESIA FOR
THORACIC SURGERY

Dedicated to my family,
Glynis, Ben & Polly

ANAESTHESIA FOR THORACIC SURGERY

J.W.W.GOTHARD

MB BS FFARCS
Consultant Anaesthetist
Royal Brompton
National Heart and Lung Hospital
London

WITH A CONTRIBUTION BY
BEVERLY A. SUTTON

FCAnaes SRN
Senior Registrar in Anaesthesia
St George's Hospital
London

SECOND EDITION

OXFORD
BLACKWELL SCIENTIFIC PUBLICATIONS
LONDON EDINBURGH BOSTON
MELBOURNE PARIS BERLIN VIENNA

© 1982, 1993 by
Blackwell Scientific Publications
Editorial Offices:
Osney Mead, Oxford OX2 0EL
25 John Street, London WC1N 2BL
23 Ainslie Place, Edinburgh EH3 6AJ
238 Main Street, Cambridge
  Massachusetts 02142, USA
54 University Street, Carlton
  Victoria 3053, Australia

Other Editorial Offices:
Librairie Arnette SA
2, rue Casimir-Delavigne
75006 Paris
France

Blackwell Wissenschafts-Verlag GmbH
Meinekestrasse 4
D-1000 Berlin 15
Germany

Blackwell MZV
Feldgasse 13
A-1238 Wien
Austria

First published 1982
Second edition 1993

Set by Semantic Graphics, Singapore
Printed and bound in Great Britain
at the University Press, Cambridge

DISTRIBUTORS

Marston Book Services Ltd
PO Box 87
Oxford OX2 0DT
(*Orders*: Tel: 0865 791155
        Fax: 0865 791927
        Telex: 837515)

USA
Blackwell Scientific Publications, Inc.
238 Main Street
Cambridge, MA 02142
(*Orders*: Tel: 800 759-6102
        617 876-7000)

Canada
Times Mirror Professional Publishing, Ltd
130 Flaska Drive
Markham, Ontario L6G 1B8
(*Orders*: Tel: 800 268-4178
        416 470-6739)

Australia
Blackwell Scientific Publications Pty Ltd
54 University Street
Carlton, Victoria 3053
(*Orders*: Tel: 03 347-5552)

A catalogue record for this title
is available from the British Library

ISBN 0-632-03275-8

Library of Congress
Cataloging-in-Publication Data

Gothard, J.W.W.
    Anaesthesia for thoracic surgery/
  J.W.W. Gothard; with a contribution by
  Beverly A. Sutton. — 2nd ed.
        p.   cm.
    Includes bibliographical references and
  index.
      1. Chest—Surgery.   2. Anesthesia.
  I. Sutton, Beverly A.   II. Title
    [DNLM: 1. Anesthesia.   2. Thoracic
  Surgery.   WF 980 G684a]
  RD536.G63   1993
  617.9′6754—dc20

Contents

Preface to the Second Edition

It is now over 10 years since Margaret Branthwaite and I wrote the first edition of *Anaesthesia for Thoracic Surgery*. There have been significant changes in the practice of thoracic anaesthesia during this time and the addition of a considerable amount of material to the literature.

This second edition, as before, covers all forms of adult, non-cardiac thoracic surgery. The text is directed primarily at anaesthetists in training but the specialist anaesthetist will find the new and revised sections, including those on endobronchial intubation, one-lung anaesthesia, mediastinal tumours and lung transplantation, of considerable interest. There are over 50 new illustrations in the book and Dr Beverly Sutton has contributed an excellent, entirely new, chapter on postoperative management with emphasis on postoperative pain relief. In addition, the reference sections have been completely revised and updated.

I am grateful for the technical support I have received from Dr Stuart Taylor of Blackwell Scientific Publications and from both the Photographic and Medical Illustration Departments of the Royal Marsden Hospital. I am indebted to many colleagues at the Royal Brompton Hospital for their help and advice over the last 15 years. Thanks are particularly due to Mr Peter Goldstraw, Consultant Thoracic Surgeon, whose surgical skill and enthusiasm has continued to stimulate my interest in the clinical practice of thoracic anaesthesia. Finally, I would like to acknowledge my sincere gratitude to Dr Margaret Branthwaite. She first encouraged my interest in medical writing and was tremendously supportive to me in my early career, as she was to many young anaesthetists.

London   John W.W. Gothard

Preface to the First Edition

O! what men dare do!
What men may do!
What men daily do, not knowing
what they do!

Much Ado About Nothing iv.1

The foundations of modern cardiothoracic anaesthesia were established in the first half of this century when techniques, concepts and apparatus were developed which have transformed procedures once regarded as hazardous into the straightforward routine of today. It is tempting, and indeed perhaps conventional, to discuss the historical background to current practice in some detail but, important though this era was, we have chosen to review only briefly those procedures, methods and items of equipment which are no longer widely used.

We have attempted instead to provide an account of anaesthesia for all forms of elective, non-cardiac thoracic surgery as it is practised today, and our text is directed primarily to postgraduates training in anaesthesia and preparing for higher examinations. We have described methods in use at the Brompton Hospital but recognize that alternatives exist, and so we have tried to explain, wherever possible, those theoretical and practical factors which must be understood clearly because they form the logical basis for choosing a technique which will be both safe and effective.

We are indebted to many of our colleagues for helpful discussion and advice, particularly Mr P. Goldstraw, Consultant Thoracic Surgeon, who has commented on many of the surgical aspects, and Dr M.J.H. Scallan, Consultant Anaesthetist, who has given us the benefit of his expertise in paediatric anaesthesia. Our warmest thanks go to Dr I.C.W. English, Senior Anaesthetist at the Brompton Hospital. He has taught us both, his practical skills have stimulated our enthusiasm and he has given us unceasing encouragement. We appreciate his generous foreword and it is a pleasure to place on record the gratitude, affection and respect felt for him by a long series of his trainees.

London 1981
J.W.W. Gothard
M.A. Branthwaite

1: History

THE DEVELOPMENT OF THORACIC SURGERY

Major developments in both thoracic surgery and anaesthesia have occurred during the 20th century and it is instructive to consider how current practice has evolved throughout these years.

Empyema and tuberculosis were the main indications for thoracic surgery at the beginning of the century. The former was treated by rib resection and drainage and the latter primarily by collapse of the lung. This was usually achieved by creating an artificial pneumothorax, but a number of patients required division of adhesions so that the lung could retract, and some were selected for the more aggressive treatment of phrenic nerve avulsion. Thoracoplasty was introduced to the UK by Morriston Davies in 1912 but was considered hazardous at first and so was performed infrequently. The procedure gained in popularity between the two World Wars as both experience and expertise were acquired, and occasional thoracotomies were also performed for lung resection and the removal of tumours using a snare or tourniquet technique. The first successful pneumonectomy was carried out for bronchiectasis by Nissen in Germany in 1931. Techniques for dissecting and ligating individual structures at the hilum of the lung were soon developed and, combined with an improved understanding of the disturbances created by opening the pleural cavity, led to an increasing interest in pulmonary resection.

Experience in the management of chest wounds, gained during World War II by teams of thoracic surgeons and anaesthetists, the more widespread use of blood transfusion, and the introduction of sulphonamides by May and Baker in 1938, all increased the chances of survival after thoracic surgery or injury.

1

The treatment of infective lung disease was revolutionized in the postwar period by the availability of penicillin for civilian use and the discovery of streptomycin (1943), *para*-aminosalicylic acid (1946) and isoniazid (1952). Pulmonary tuberculosis and bronchiectasis were treated surgically less and less often, whereas resection for malignant disease became more common, a trend which has continued to the present time. Primary carcinoma of the bronchus is probably now the most common indication for thoracotomy in the UK, but carcinoma of the oesophagus, resection for metastatic disease after the successful treatment of an extrathoracic primary tumour, as well as a variety of benign conditions also feature prominently in the thoracic surgeon's practice.

PROGRESS IN ANAESTHESIA

Many of these developments would have been impossible without simultaneous advances in anaesthesia. The most important have been: the use of endotracheal and, subsequently, endobronchial intubation; the introduction of muscle relaxants; and the increasing popularity and sophistication of techniques of controlled ventilation. As a result, the risks of asphyxia or spread of disease by the dissemination of infected secretions, the hazards associated with spontaneous ventilation when one hemithorax is open, and the consequences of using deep general anaesthesia to inhibit coughing and straining during manipulation of the thoracic viscera have virtually all been eliminated.

Management of the airway and control of secretions

Contemporary endotracheal anaesthesia owes much to the pioneering work of Rowbotham and Magill which was prompted by the need to provide safe operating conditions for maxillo-facial surgery in servicemen injured during World War I. In spite of his own remarkable skill at both blind nasal and orotracheal intubation, Magill expressed the following view as late as 1928 in a communication to the Anaesthetic Section of the Royal Society of Medicine: 'Operations on the thorax, such as thoracoplasty and pulmonary decortication, give better results when nitrous oxide or ethylene and oxygen are administered by means of a facepiece. The condition of the patient after operation is ample compensation for the difficulty sometimes entailed in maintaining airtight apposition of the mask. Moreover, an efficient apparatus provides for positive ventilation of the lungs without the necessity for intubation.'

However, it was only a year or two after this that Gale and Waters in the US, and Magill himself in the UK, popularized endobronchial intubation and one-lung anaesthesia for thoracic surgery.

Techniques of endobronchial blocking were described about the same time by Magill in 1934 and Crafoord in 1938 and were intended to exclude the operated lobe or lung from tidal ventilation and to retain secretions within it. Double-lumen tubes are a later development, usually regarded as derivatives of the Carlens' catheter which was introduced in 1949 for differential bronchospirometry. As with so many apparent innovations, the same concept had been advocated previously by both Head and Frenckner, but many 'firsts' have been forgotten or discarded as a result of contemporary criticism so that the date of introduction of new techniques or apparatus is often controversial. Many of the endobronchial tubes introduced in the 1950s are now no longer manufactured (Tables 1.1–1.3). The most popular double-lumen tubes are now disposable and follow on from the introduction of the Bronchocath tube (Mallinckrodt, National Catheter Corporation) in 1982, although Phoenix Medical Ltd now manufacture the highly successful, original-pattern, Robertshaw tube in both reusable and disposable forms.

An alternative to endobronchial instrumentation for the control of secretions during thoracic surgery has been the use of posture. Beecher

Table 1.1 Bronchus blockers and combinations of historical interest

Bronchus blockers
Magill, 1934
A suction catheter with a streamlined cuff. Small enough to pass down the lumen of an 8 mm bronchoscope or lie within an endotracheal tube. A wire stylette was used to stiffen the catheter during placement.

Crafoord, 1938
Crafoord blocked bronchi with a ribbon gauze tampon inserted directly via a bronchoscope. Tracheal intubation was used in conjunction with this technique.

Vernon–Thompson, 1943
Larger than the Magill device, this blocker also had a wire stylette to aid placement. The rubber balloon had a distinctive gauze mesh cover to prevent overdistension and movement once in place. It was most suitable for use in the left main bronchus.

Combination of an endotracheal tube and a bronchus blocker
Stürtzbecher, 1953
The combination of an endotracheal tube and bronchus blocker, with a wire stylette to aid blind placement.

Macintosh–Leatherdale, 1955
Shaped combination of an endotracheal tube and left-sided bronchus blocker (Fig. 1.3).

Table 1.2 Single-lumen endobronchial tubes of historical interest

---

Gale and Waters, 1932
A single-lumen tube with detachable carinal cuff. The tube was inserted blindly into one main bronchus and the cuff inflated to exclude the other bronchus.

Magill, 1936
A single-lumen tube made of rubber over an inner wire spiral. This was inserted over an intubating bronchoscope. A later development was the right-sided tube with the wire spiral beyond the cuff left bare to prevent obstruction of the right upper lobe orifice (Fig. 1.4).

Gordon–Green, 1955
A right-sided tube with tracheal and bronchial cuffs. The original tube was inserted blindly and located with the aid of the angulated endobronchial portion of the tube and a carinal hook. The carinal hook was often removed and the tube inserted under direct vision using an intubating bronchoscope (Fig. 1.5).

Macintosh–Leatherdale, 1955
Shaped tube for blind placement in the left main bronchus.

Brompton–Pallister, 1959
Triple-cuffed tube, with double bronchial cuff, for bronchoscopic placement in the left main bronchus. Originally designed for sleeve resection of the right upper lobe.

(1940) recognized that a steep head-down tilt in the lateral position would favour drainage rather than soiling of the dependent lung whereas Overholt (1946), also working in the US, used the prone position to retain secretions in the diseased areas (Fig. 1.1). In the UK, Parry Brown (1948) popularized pulmonary resection in a prone position which allowed free drainage of secretions without soiling and without an extreme head-down tilt (Fig. 1.2). The surgical technique is very different with the patient prone and very few surgeons are now familiar with this approach.

Regional anaesthesia was advocated at one time as a means of preventing the spread of secretions because it was thought that the cough reflex would

Table 1.3 Double-lumen endobronchial tubes of historical interest

---

Carlens, 1950
A left-sided double-lumen tube with carinal hook, originally introduced for differential bronchospirometry in 1949. Still used in some centres (Fig. 1.6).

White, 1960
Right-sided version of the Carlens' tube with a ventilation slot in the bronchial cuff for right upper lobe ventilation.

Bryce–Smith, 1959 and Bryce–Smith and Salt, 1960
Tubes for left and right endobronchial intubation respectively.

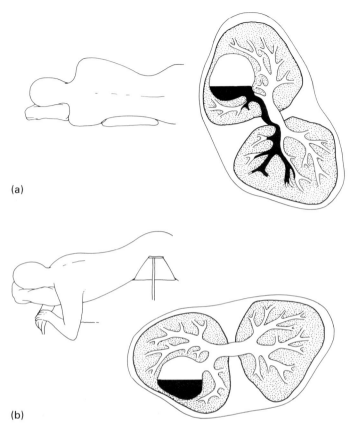

Fig. 1.1 Cross-section of the thorax showing (a) that secretions drain from the upper lung in the lateral position but (b) are retained in the dependent lung in the Overholt position.

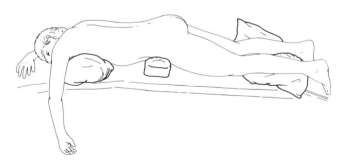

Fig. 1.2 Parry Brown, prone thoracotomy position.

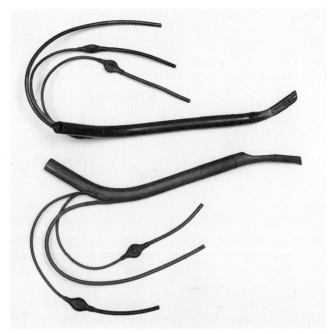

Fig. 1.3 Macintosh–Leatherdale combined endotracheal tube and left bronchial blocker, seen from above the from the side.

be retained. This belief was questioned in the early 1940s when it was realized that coughing is ineffective in the lateral position with an open hemithorax, and is more likely to spread infection than control it. However,

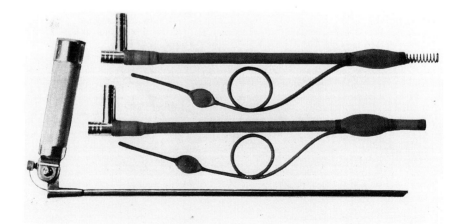

Fig. 1.4 Magill's right and left endobronchial tubes and intubating bronchoscope.

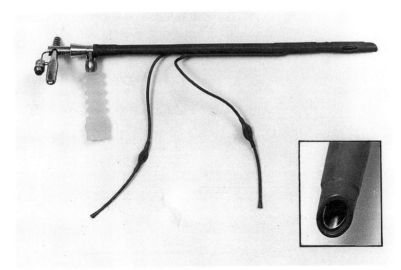

Fig. 1.5 A Gordon–Green single-lumen right endobronchial tube mounted on an intubating bronchoscope. *Inset.* The bevels of the tube and bronchoscope are aligned.

regional techniques remained popular for thoracoplasty, particularly para-vertebral block with local infiltration.

Control of ventilation

Collapse of healthy, non-adherent lung is inevitable when one pleural cavity

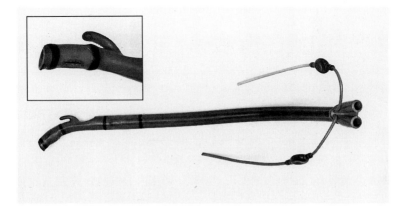

Fig. 1.6 Carlens' left double-lumen tube. *Inset* shows distal end of a White tube.

is opened widely to atmospheric pressure in a spontaneously breathing subject.

As early as 1904, Ferdinand Sauerbruch published the results of his studies on lung collapse during thoracotomy in man and concluded that it was necessary to create a differential pressure across the lungs to keep them inflated. He advocated the use of an operating chamber in which the patient's chest (and the surgical team) were maintained at a negative pressure. The chamber was sealed around the patient's neck, so permitting spontaneous respiration at ambient pressure. An alternative and more practical technique was suggested by Brauer, a colleague of Sauerbruch, who delivered compressed air and anaesthetic gases to a positive pressure box placed around the patient's head. Positive pressure breathing methods of this type were popular for a number of years and a catalogue from Drager included such an apparatus as recently as 1948. Hypercapnia was soon recognized as a complication of these methods, and rhythmic pressure or inflation at infrequent but regular intervals was sometimes used to control it.

Insufflation of gases into the trachea was an alternative, described at about the same time in the US by Meltzer and Auer who demonstrated that satisfactory gas exchange can be achieved if gas is blown under pressure into the trachea through a narrow catheter and allowed to escape around it. The technique renders the patient virtually apnoeic and was popular for thoracic surgery in the US for a number of years. A modern derivative is the insufflation of gases during bronchoscopy, now largely superseded by the injector technique introduced by Sanders in 1967. There has been little enthusiasm for insufflation for pulmonary surgery in the UK but it was advocated for surgery on the head, neck and upper air passages because the outflow of gas around the endotracheal catheter helped to prevent blood and debris soiling the lungs.

Delivery of gases to the lungs by positive pressure through an endotracheal tube or tracheostomy has been recognized for centuries as a method of resuscitation but has been accepted during anaesthesia only relatively recently. The advent of cyclopropane and subsequent introduction of muscle relaxants facilitated the development of assisted and then controlled ventilation in the 1930s and 1940s by Waters in the US and Nosworthy in the UK. At first, ventilation was carried out by manual compression of a bag in a closed circuit system which included a soda lime canister to ensure carbon dioxide removal. A mechanical device for assisting inspiration via an endotracheal catheter had been described by Janeway in 1913 and an early ventilator, the Spiropulsator, was designed by Frenckner in 1934. Crafoord's modification of the Spiropulsator was introduced in 1938 and soon used widely in Sweden during thoracic surgery although elsewhere manual ventilation was preferred until the 1950s and later.

Fully controlled ventilation of the lungs using light general anaesthesia and muscular relaxation has eliminated the need for deep inhalational anaesthesia, with its risks of respiratory or cardiovascular depression during or after surgery. It does, however, introduce the possibility of inadequate suppression of humoral and autonomic responses to stress and also of awareness during surgery.

FURTHER READING

Holmes Sellors T. (1975) Half a century of thoracic surgery. *Journal of the Irish Colleges of Physicians and Surgeons*, **5**, 26–30.

Magill I.W. (1978) Endotracheal anaesthesia. Reprinted from *Proceedings of the Royal Society of Medicine* 1929; xxii: 83. *Anaesthesia*, **33**, 580–586.

Meade R.H. (1961) *A History of Thoracic Surgery*. Charles C. Thomas, Springfield, Illinois.

Mushin W.W. & Rendell-Baker L. (1953) *The Principles of Thoracic Anaesthesia Past and Present*. Blackwell Scientific Publications, Oxford.

Paraskevopoulos J.A., Gunning A.J. & Dennison A.R. (1991) The changing pattern of thoracic surgery in the United Kingdom 1963–1982. *Journal of the Royal Society of Medicine*, **84**, 484–487.

White G.M.J. (1960) Evolution of endotracheal and endobronchial intubation. *British Journal of Anaesthesia*, **32**, 235–246.

2: Preoperative Considerations

Preoperative assessment should aim to fulfil three objectives. The first is to understand the implications of the disease for which surgery has been recommended and the consequences of the procedure which is planned. The second is to confirm that optimum preoperative preparation has been achieved, and the third is to recognize and make allowance for any coexistent disease or idiosyncrasy of physique or personality. The implications of specific conditions and procedures encountered in thoracic surgery are dealt with individually in subsequent chapters; the consequences of extrathoracic disease, allergy, drug therapy and individual personal characteristics are common to all forms of surgery and are not considered here. This chapter aims instead to highlight those anatomical and functional features which are of particular relevance to non-cardiac thoracic surgery, and to outline preoperative measures which can be used to create the best possible conditions for a successful outcome.

COMMON SYMPTOMS AND THEIR SIGNIFICANCE

Dyspnoea

This is a subjective symptom, notoriously unreliable as a test of functional

10

capacity until it is extreme. Quite marked loss of pulmonary function occurring gradually in a sedentary subject may be ignored or even denied, whereas the previously healthy and active often complain bitterly about minor degrees of exercise limitation. Enquiry about the ability to sustain specific levels of effort is very much more accurate than 'Are you ever short of breath?'. Alternatively, a simple exercise test can be carried out, for example, can the patient walk briskly up two flights of stairs while maintaining a conversation? What distance can the patient walk in 6 or 12 minutes and does he or she appear short of breath or have an undue tachycardia after the test?

Dyspnoea in those presenting for thoracic surgery usually indicates disease of the lungs or airway but other causes must be remembered too. Possibilities include unrecognized cardiac disease, anaemia and deformity or rigidity of the thoracic cage. It is particularly important to recognize dyspnoea caused by an obstructive lesion of the trachea or main bronchi. Although sometimes amenable to complete relief by surgery, obstruction at these sites can interfere with control of the airway during induction, with intubation, with the distribution of gas during mechanical ventilation and with respiratory function in the immediate postoperative period. Superior vena caval obstruction is another cause of dyspnoea with specific implications for the anaesthetist (see Chapter 10) and may be present in association with a lesion of the proximal tracheobronchial tree.

Much more commonly, dyspnoea signifies disease of the peripheral airways or of the alveoli. Spasm, mucosal oedema and obstruction by mucus interfere with gas flow, as does premature closure of small airways during expiration, because of reduced elastic recoil. Dyspnoea caused by disease of the small airways is frequently accompanied by wheezing and is often very variable in severity, especially in patients with asthma and, to a lesser extent, those with chronic bronchitis. This is a particularly important feature to note at the preoperative visit because a variety of anaesthetic drugs as well as instrumentation within the respiratory tract are likely to precipitate an abrupt and sometimes life-threatening increase in airway resistance. By contrast, dyspnoea caused by generalized lung disease at the level of the alveoli (e.g. infiltration or fibrosis) is unlikely to change on a moment-to-moment basis, although it has been suggested that deterioration over a period of days can follow exposure to high concentrations of oxygen in the operative or postoperative period when pulmonary damage is caused by certain cytotoxic drugs (e.g. bleomycin) or some types of fibrosis.

Dyspnoea is usually not a prominent symptom of those operated on for an isolated lesion within one lobe or lung. Exceptions are those patients with air-filled cysts or bullae (see Chapter 7) and those in whom an inflammatory lesion is accompanied by an excess of secretions within the respiratory tract. Patients who are short of breath at rest warrant particularly careful assessment. The cause is usually obvious and the important requirement is to ascertain whether some specific treatment, such as the insertion of a chest drain, can improve pulmonary function before surgery.

Cough and the production of sputum

The presence of a dry cough is of little practical importance although it often indicates an irritative lesion of the trachea or main bronchi, or compression by glands. Its abolition may necessitate a deeper level of anaesthesia than might otherwise be necessary, but is unlikely to have any other effect on the course or conduct of the anaesthetic. The presence of a productive cough is far more noteworthy. Secretions are likely to spread during operation, interfering with the airway at the time and increasing the risk of collapse and infection later. An early morning cough resulting in the expectoration of a small amount of mucoid sputum is regarded as 'normal' by most smokers and many of those who suffer from chronic sinusitis with a nocturnal postnasal drip. The question 'Do you have a cough or produce any sputum?' often elicits a negative answer from such patients unless they are questioned closely about symptoms at this time of day.

Haemoptysis

This is a common symptom of many inflammatory and neoplastic diseases of the lung and is usually minor — no more than blood-streaking of the sputum. Large haemoptyses are less common and are associated particularly with bronchiectasis, aspergillomata and cavitating tuberculosis. Haemoptysis is sometimes a prominent symptom of vascular tumours or malformations but massive bleeding is unusual unless the tumour has been biopsied.

A history of minor haemoptysis does not usually influence anaesthetic management but an episode of severe bleeding means that some form of isolation technique should be used during surgery.

Dysphagia

It is important to distinguish between true dysphagia — an inability to swallow — and reluctance to swallow because of pain. Patients who are unable to swallow soon become cachectic and dehydrated with the result that, if the obstruction is chronic, the oesophagus dilates and may contain food residues. These might be infected and may spill into the airway during anaesthesia. Pain immediately after swallowing is common in patients with reflux oesophagitis and the presence of this symptom warrants efforts to reduce gastric acidity preoperatively and to protect the airway during induction of anaesthesia.

PHYSICAL EXAMINATION

The general build of the patient is noted and particular attention is paid to height, the configuration of the jaw and the state of the teeth. Patients who are unduly tall or short for their age and sex may be difficult to intubate with non-disposable double-lumen tubes which are designed to fit the 'average' length trachea of a particular diameter. Disposable double-lumen tubes are, in general, longer and less bulky but their final position may need checking with the fibreoptic bronchoscope (see Chapter 5). Endobronchial tubes are less easy to manipulate than endotracheal tubes but the facial characteristics which suggest that difficulty may be experienced are similar for both. Prominent or loose teeth and gaps in the dentition of the upper jaw are likely to interfere with rigid bronchoscopy, oesophagoscopy or any form of endobronchial instrumentation. Dental caps and crowns on upper incisors are easily damaged and particularly vulnerable during the passage of a rigid, straight bronchoscope or oesophagoscope.

The need for endobronchial instrumentation should also prompt careful examination of the position and direction of the trachea and, while examining the neck, the height of the venous pressure, the presence or absence of collateral vessels and the degree of swelling and superficial engorgement can be observed in those with superior caval obstruction. Cyanosis in the distribution of superior caval drainage is common when the vessel is obstructed, whereas central cyanosis suggests that there is either generalized disease of the lungs or airways, or a large area of collapse or consolidation.

Chest wall movement is often asymmetric in patients requiring surgery for pulmonary disease and is impaired if an intercostal drain is in place. Most attention should be paid to the mobility and excursion of the healthy side but, if a chest drain is in place, the use of suction should be noted as well as the magnitude of the respiratory swing or the volume of air escaping through the underwater seal. Stridor resulting from a tracheal lesion is often audible at a distance but auscultation is necessary to detect the fixed, single pitch rhonchus caused by a partially obstructed main or lobar bronchus. Rhonchi throughout both lung fields are characteristic of generalized airway obstruction but sometimes can only be detected on forced expiration. Coarse râles influenced in their location by coughing suggest loose secretions within the bronchial tree, whereas those signifying disease of the peripheral airways or alveoli are usually more constant and less obtrusive.

The examination concludes with an assessment of the cardiovascular system and of any other physical characteristics which may be relevant in individual cases; for example, severe arthritis or skeletal deformity. It should be remembered that many of the patients presenting with carcinoma of the bronchus will be elderly life-long smokers and are therefore likely to have significant cardiovascular disease. This aspect of the preoperative assessment and its impact on the risks of surgery are discussed in more detail below.

PREOPERATIVE INVESTIGATION

A full blood count, urine test, electrocardiogram (ECG), and the measurement of blood glucose and urea and electrolyte concentrations are carried out routinely. A recent chest X-ray and baseline lung function tests should also be available. Liver function and blood coagulation tests may be appropriate in specific circumstances, particularly in those patients scheduled for major oesophageal surgery. Liver and bone scans will usually have been carried out to exclude secondary deposits in patients with malignant disease.

It is usual to crossmatch 3–4 units of blood to cover a lung resection, but in patients with a normal preoperative haemoglobin level it is often possible to avoid transfusion of blood products altogether. The use of autologous blood transfusion would not appear to be a priority in patients with lung cancer.

RADIOLOGY

Inspection of a postero-anterior and lateral chest X-ray will demonstrate the site of any localized lesion and its relationship to the hilum, mediastinum and chest wall. The direction, shape and diameter of the trachea and main bronchi can often be determined from these films, and this may alert the anaesthetist to potential problems with endobronchial intubation (Fig. 2.1). Enhanced digital chest radiography may be particularly useful in delineating the airways and apical pneumothoraces. It is also possible in many cases to identify the interlobar fissures and hence predict whether distortion of the bronchial tree below the carina is likely. Evidence of previous disease may be apparent; for example, healed or calcified tuberculous foci or a past episode of pleurisy. The latter is worthy of note because it suggests there may be adhesions which sometimes cause troublesome haemorrhage during dissection. The volume of the lungs, contour of the diaphragm, and the density and

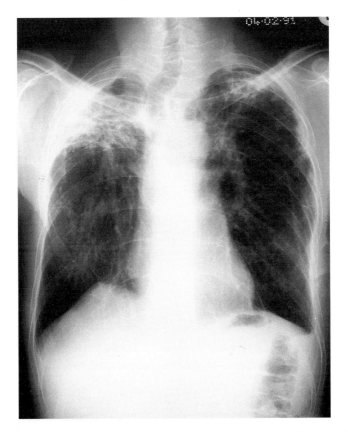

Fig. 2.1 The preoperative chest X-ray of an adult male patient. Bilateral apical scarring, more extensive on the right side, has caused distortion of the trachea. Endobronchial intubation was achieved at operation using a fibreoptic bronchoscope to place the tube under direct vision.

uniformity of lung markings are often abnormal in patients with emphysema and, particularly in the elderly, a rather large heart and unfolded aorta suggest that the cardiovascular system may be non-compliant and so respond poorly to surgical stress.

Often more than one imaging technique will be required to assess the extent of intrathoracic disease and its operability (Figs 2.2–2.4). These are discussed below.

Tomography

The conventional chest radiograph is a two-dimensional image of a three-dimensional structure. Images from the entire depth of the chest are

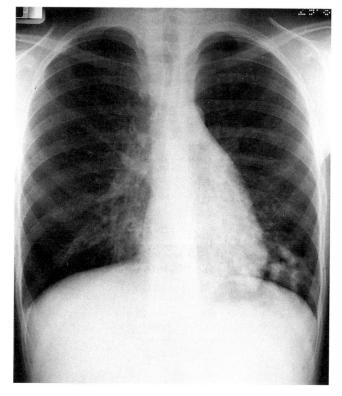

Fig. 2.2 Chest X-ray of a 10-year-old boy with left lower lobe consolidation.

superimposed on one another, interfering with the detection and delineation of such features as small lesions or cavities, hilar glands, the vascular connections of a tumour, or the precise shape and disposition of the mediastinal structures (particularly the trachea and main bronchi). Structures in one plane only are in focus in a tomogram and it was customary to expose a series of films, usually at 1 cm intervals, so that a three-dimensional image of the structure in question could be visualized. The use of computerized tomography scanning (CT scanning) and magnetic resonance imaging (MRI) has largely superseded the simpler tomographic techniques.

Computerized tomography scanning and magnetic resonance imaging

Computerized tomography and faster Imatron scanning techniques are now an established method of demonstrating lesions within the thorax which

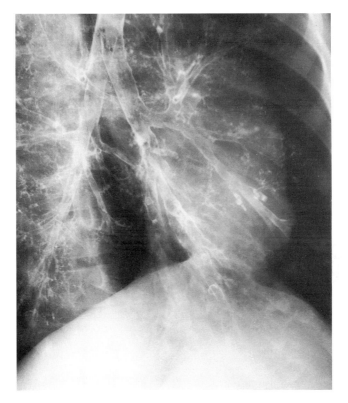

Fig. 2.3 A bronchogram on the same patient as in Fig. 2.2 demonstrates abnormally dilated bronchi in the lingula and left lower lobe.

cannot be easily demonstrated by conventional radiology. CT scanning is used to identify the site, size and possible extension of intrathoracic tumours originating in the lungs and mediastinum. Airway pathology can also be delineated quite clearly. Patients with primary lung cancer are accepted for surgery if there is no evidence of nodal spread on a CT scan. Those with mediastinal lymphadenopathy will still require mediastinoscopy and biopsy of the nodes for accurate staging because previous infective conditions and reactive hyperplasia of the tumour can cause appearances identical to that of malignant enlargement.

MRI has not proven superior to CT scanning for the investigation of intrathoracic pathology except for the delineation of vascular structures. MRI can be used to identify the site and extent of aortic dissection and may also be useful in imaging tumour invasion of the heart.

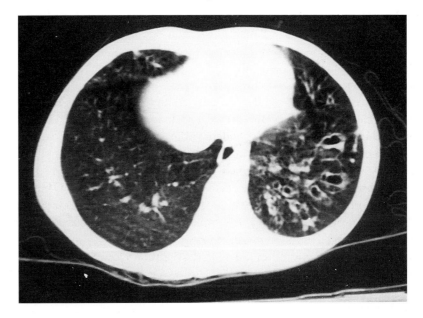

Fig. 2.4 A CT scan of the thorax clearly demonstrates grossly dilated bronchi in the left lung (same patient as in Figs 2.2 and 2.3).

Other imaging techniques

CT scans can be 'enhanced' with intravenous contrast medium and bronchography is used to outline the tracheobronchial tree by the instillation of radio-opaque dye (Fig. 2.3). This latter investigation is of particular value in the management of patients with bronchiectasis and is described in more detail in Chapter 3.

Radioisotope scans of both lungs in the postero-anterior and lateral planes are used to observe the distribution of ventilation and perfusion and, in the context of thoracic surgery, are of most value in the investigation of regional lung function.

ASSESSMENT OF PULMONARY FUNCTION

Spirometry and the flow–volume loop

Many patients are accepted for thoracic surgery without formal measurements of pulmonary function. There is no reason to dispute this practice in those with a localized lesion and no past or present history of pulmonary disease. On the other hand, bedside measurements of vital capacity (VC), forced expired volume in one second (FEV_1) and peak expiratory flow rate (PEFR) are so easy to record that they could sensibly be carried out as a routine. They should, in any case, be regarded as the bare minimum in patients with a history of dyspnoea or chronic productive cough, or those who are heavy, life-long smokers. Values of 1 and 2 litres respectively for FEV_1 and forced vital capacity (FVC) are often quoted as the lower limit which can be accepted before pneumonectomy. However, these arbitrary values allow neither for size- and age-dependent variation in predicted normal values, nor for the fact that a reduced VC may reflect disease confined to the operated side rather than uniform impairment of function throughout both lungs.

Both obstructive and restrictive defects cause a reduction in VC but there is a disproportionate fall in the FEV_1 in those with airway obstruction, whilst in those with a restrictive defect, the ratio of FEV_1 to FVC is normal or high. In general, changes in PEFR parallel those in the FEV_1/FVC ratio. A PEFR of less than 70% of predicted or an FEV_1/FVC ratio below 60% are adverse features in patients requiring pulmonary surgery. More information can be obtained if the forced expiratory manoeuvre is recorded so that flow rate is plotted against volume; this is known as the flow–volume loop (Fig. 2.5). In those with airflow limitation associated with asthma or bronchitis, there is usually a marked volume-dependent reduction in expiratory flow rate but inspiratory flow is less affected. In patients with emphysema, airflow limitation is more markedly pressure dependent; thus emphysematous patients can also exhale a greater volume as a relaxed VC manoeuvre than when expiration is forced. If expiratory airflow limitation is detected, it is worth repeating the test after the supervised inhalation of a bronchodilator such as 200 µg of salbutamol. Reversibility is judged to be present when this results in improvement by at least 20% in one or more of these indices. Although this confirms therapeutic responsiveness, airway obstruction which reverses easily can also deteriorate equally easily, sometimes making management during anaesthesia and mechanical ventilation more difficult than when airway obstruction is irreversible. It is also worth noting that mechanical ventilation is often surprisingly easy when pressure-dependent airway closure is the sole mechanism of obstruction, as in a proportion of patients with emphysema.

A central obstructive lesion (e.g. in the trachea) causes a fall in inspiratory as well as expiratory flow rate, but restrictive defects such as rigidity of the chest wall or a thickened pleura, or diaphragmatic paralysis, cannot be distinguished from central obstruction on the basis of the flow–volume loop alone.

Maximum breathing capacity (MBC) or maximum voluntary ventilation is a value which has achieved some popularity as a means of identifying

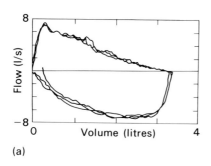

(a)

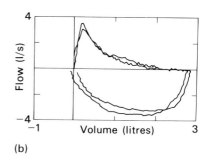

(b)

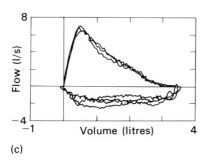

(c)

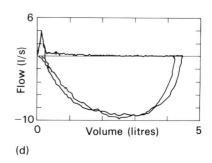

(d)

Fig. 2.5 Flow–volume loops. (a) Normal, (b) volume-dependent airway collapse, (c) tracheal obstruction from a mediastinal tumour, (d) pressure-dependent airway collapse. Note the different scales.

patients at risk of pulmonary insufficiency after resection. It is determined during a period of voluntary hyperventilation for 15 s through a low resistance circuit. A value of 40 litres/min or 20 litres/min m^2 of body surface area, corresponding to an FEV_1 of approximately 1 litre after resection, is widely regarded as a threshold below which the risks of respiratory failure following pulmonary resection are unacceptable. Formerly calculated on the basis of functional losses of approximately 25% after lobectomy or 33% after pneumonectomy, and disregarding the nature of location of the lesion, these predictions can now be made with far greater accuracy using preoperative radiospirometry in which the distribution of ventilation and perfusion is assessed on a regional basis.

Measurements of lung volume and gas transfer

Total lung capacity can be determined in a number of ways: whole body plethysmography, helium dilution or a quantitative analysis of postero-anterior and lateral chest X-rays. The difference between total lung capacity as measured by plethysmography and an inert gas dilution technique is used as an index of air trapping.

Ventilation and perfusion can be studied by inhaling or injecting labelled xenon or krypton, and these techniques are amenable to quantitation so that it is possible to predict, preoperatively, values for postoperative VC, FEV_1 and MBC. These are calculated from the preoperative value for each variable, multiplied by the proportion of lung which will remain as determined from the preoperative scan; predictions based solely on perfusion scans appear as reliable as those where both ventilation and perfusion are studied. Measurements can be performed at rest and on exercise; information derived from the latter may be of most prognostic value. The use of MBC to define the lower limit of operability has received renewed interest now that it is possible to predict whether the threshold value of 20 litres/min/m^2 body surface area (corresponding to an FEV_1 of about 0.8–1.0 litre) will be attained postoperatively, after resection of lung which is contributing to the value measured preoperatively.

Another method of evaluating operability is based on the realization that pulmonary hypertension and right ventricular failure contribute to mortality and morbidity in some patients, particularly those requiring pneumonectomy. Attempts have been made to predict inoperability on the basis of changes in pulmonary arterial pressure at rest, on exercise, and in the same circumstances after balloon occlusion of the pulmonary artery on the diseased side. Table 2.1 enumerates criteria which have been suggested to identify patients in whom postoperative mortality will be high. These measurements add very considerably to the cost, complexity and risk of preoperative evaluation and, because they do not discriminate with sufficient

Table 2.1 Summary from Baier (1980) of criteria based on the assessment of pulmonary vascular function which have been associated with an increased mortality after pulmonary resection

Mean PAP at rest	> 22–30 mmHg
Mean PAP at rest on balloon occlusion	> 26–32 mmHg
Mean PAP during exercise on balloon occlusion	> 35 mmHg
Systemic PaO_2 during exercise on balloon occlusion	< 6.00 kPa (45 mmHg)

PAP, pulmonary arterial pressure

reliability between operable and inoperable cases, they have not gained widespread acceptance. Measurement of pulmonary arterial pressure at the time of operation during balloon occlusion on the operated side is a compromise but is of no value as a means of identifying patients who should not be subjected to thoracotomy at all.

Exercise testing and lung resection

Formal exercise testing on the cycle ergometer may have a role to play in the evaluation of operative risk for thoracotomy. Smith *et al.* (1984) found that patients with a maximal oxygen uptake of more than 20 ml/kg/min had very few complications following thoracotomy whereas those with an oxygen uptake of less than 15 ml/kg/min had a very high incidence of postoperative problems. However, in a more recent study (Boysen *et al.*, 1990), this clear-cut distinction was not confirmed. These conflicting findings have been discussed by Fishman and Systrom (1991).

ASSESSMENT OF CARDIAC FUNCTION

As previously stated, many patients with lung cancer are elderly, life-long smokers. Cardiorespiratory dysfunction is the major cause of death following lung resection and therefore particular attention must be paid to the patient's cardiovascular status, in addition to pulmonary function. A detailed history, clinical examination, chest X-ray and ECG will reveal many cardiac abnormalities, including ischaemia, cardiac failure and valve disease. Special investigations such as exercise testing, echocardiography and angiography may also be indicated. Drug therapy for angina, cardiac failure and dysrhythmias should be instituted where appropriate and administered up to the time of surgery.

Outcome studies of intraoperative predictors have shown that prolonged thoracic surgery is associated with an increased risk of cardiac morbidity. Goldman's Multifactorial Index of Cardiac Risk in Non-Cardiac Surgery encompasses many of the factors that need to be considered in the preoperative period (Table 2.2). It is worthwhile considering such a scoring system to evaluate risk in the patient presenting for lung resection.

EVALUATING THE RISK

It might be imagined that accurate measurement of cardiopulmonary function would provide clear-cut criteria for the selection of patients who

Table 2.2 (a) Multifactorial Index of Cardiac Risk in Non-Cardiac Surgery (Goldman, 1988)

Risk factor	Points
History	
Myocardial infarction within 6 months	10
Age > 70 years	5
Physical examination	
S3 gallop or raised JVP	11
Important aortic stenosis	3
Electrocardiogram	
Rhythm other than sinus or sinus plus APB on last preoperative ECG	7
Ventricular ectopics (> 5/min)	7
Poor general medical status*	3
Intraperitoneal, intrathoracic or aortic surgery	3
Emergency operation	4

* Includes $Po_2 < 8$ kPa and $Pco_2 > 6.7$ kPa. APB, atrial premature beats; ECG, electrocardiogram; JVP, jugular venous pressure

(b) Performance of risk index in practice

Points (from above)	Life-threatening complications (%)	Cardiac deaths (%)
0–5	0.7	0.2
6–12	5	2
13–25	11	2
26 or more	22	56

would withstand pulmonary resection and would still have adequate reserves of pulmonary function postoperatively. Unfortunately, such optimism has not been borne out in practice and the 'stair climbing test' is still used as a tolerably reliable, albeit rough-and-ready, guide to fitness for surgery in uncomplicated cases. Tests of regional lung function are of considerable value as a means of judging the desirability and degree of risk in selected cases, but are by no means routine and can only be interpreted wisely in conjunction with other clinical, radiological and physiological features. It is certainly possible to identify high-risk groups on the basis of tests of pulmonary function, and criteria which should arouse anxiety are listed in Tables 2.3–2.5. However, none of these functional studies provides a reliable prognosis in individual cases.

Table 2.3 Patients fulfilling these criteria had a 56% mortality after pulmonary resection. From Didolkar *et al.* (1974)

Age ≥ 70 years
MBC ≤ 59% of predicted
Abnormal ECG

Table 2.4 Summary of criteria considered to indicate a poor prognosis after pncumonectomy. From Olsen *et al.* (1975)

FVC	< 50% predicted
FEV_1	< 50% of FVC or < 2.0 litres
MBC	< 50% predicted
RV/TLC	> 50%
T_LCO	< 50% predicted

RV/TLC, ratio of residual volume to total lung capacity; T_LCO, gas transfer

Table 2.5 Criteria identifying patients at greater-than-normal risk of morbidity or mortality postoperatively. From Tisi (1979, 1987)

MBC	< 50% predicted
FEV_1	< 2.0 litres
Pa_{CO_2}	> 6.0 kPa (45 mmHg)
Pulmonary arterial pressure during unilateral occlusion of left or right main pulmonary artery > 30 mmHg	

Other factors which influence the decision to operate include the availability of alternatives to surgery, the presence or absence of disease in other systems, and the patient's motivation and response to a discussion of the implications and risks of surgery. In UK practice a relatively high element of risk may be taken, particularly if there is a good chance of surgical cure as ascertained by preoperative staging, because resection offers the only chance of long-term survival. The final factor affecting outcome is one which can be recognized but not foreseen, namely the occurrence of operative or post-operative complications. There is certainly no easy rule or answer to the question 'Which patients will withstand lobectomy or pneumonectomy?'.

PREOPERATIVE PREPARATION

Fit patients require little preoperative preparation but all should be warned of the need for chest drains; those requiring more than minor surgery should be instructed by the physiotherapist so that they are familiar with the breathing exercises and coughing which will be required postoperatively.

Diaphragmatic breathing and lateral basal expansion are encouraged. More attention should be given to preoperative preparation of patients with poor pulmonary function, particularly if there is a treatable component to their disease such as reversible airway obstruction, chronically infected sputum or a source of re-infection in the sinuses or teeth. Those who smoke should be encouraged to stop entirely and even a short respite lessens the volume of mucus hypersecretion and hence the incidence of postoperative atelectasis and infection.

Drugs which can be used to relieve reversible airway obstruction include sympathomimetic agents, oral theophylline derivatives, ipratropium bromide (Atrovent) and inhaled corticosteroids such as beclomethasone dipropionate (Becotide). Inhaled β-sympathomimetic agents are more effective than oral preparations and some patients achieve greater benefit from a nebulized solution rather than from the pressurized aerosol. Nebulized bronchodilators such as 2.5 or 5 mg of salbutamol or terbutaline can also be administered during intermittent positive pressure ventilation (IPPV); any additional benefit in terms of bronchodilatation is, at best, only marginal but IPPV helps some patients to expectorate. Its used should be restricted to the preoperative period in those requiring pulmonary resection, because of the hazards of exposing recently completed suture lines to positive pressure.

Airway obstruction cannot be declared irreversible, even on a short-term basis, until lack of response has been demonstrated after inhaling a nebulized sympathomimetic alone and in combination with atropine. Some patients who fail to improve with these measures will respond to corticosteroids but a dose of 20–30 mg of prednisone or equivalent daily for at least 10–14 days is necessary before irreversibility can be confirmed. Those with steroid-sensitive airway obstruction will often be using the drug already and are usually given a supplement to cover anaesthesia and surgery. The maintenance dose is not increased unless essential because of possible adverse effects on wound healing and postoperative infection. However, larger doses may be required postoperatively if airway obstruction deteriorates as a result of sputum retention or infection, although measures such as inhaled sympathomimetics and infused aminophylline are usually tried first.

Patients with infected sputum should be admitted to hospital several days preoperatively so that the sputum can be cultured, appropriate antibiotics chosen, and their administration combined with regular postural drainage and chest percussion. Every effort should be made to reduce the volume of sputum and eradicate infection; this can often be achieved provided treatment is continued up to and beyond the day of operation.

Patients with severe oesophageal obstruction should be rehydrated preoperatively if there is clinical or biochemical evidence of water depletion, and a short period of intensive nutritional support is advocated by some surgeons. This can either be given parenterally or as a liquid diet infused through a small-bore nasogastric tube, if this can be introduced beyond the stricture. Attention to diet and hydration should not exclude treatment for disease in other systems and the measures outlined above for the control of common respiratory symptoms are often applicable. Patients with a hugely dilated oesophagus are sometimes prepared for surgery with repeated oesophageal lavage to remove food residues.

Prophylactic antibiotics are an issue of controversy, many surgeons electing to use them to minimize the risks of bronchial or pulmonary infection, empyema or wound abscess, whereas others withhold antibiotics prophylactically and prefer to treat postoperative infection promptly and vigorously as and when required. Specific chemotherapy must be continued in individual cases, for example patients with bronchiectasis or active tuberculosis.

The incidence of dysrhythmias complicating pneumonectomy is such that preoperative digitalization is often recommended, particularly in adult patients aged 40 years or more. Digitalization can, however, be commenced intraoperatively where indicated (see Chapter 7). Some surgical teams also cover the operation and period of greatest immobility with prophylactic heparin in low dosage to diminish the chances of pulmonary embolism without increasing the risks of operative or postoperative haemorrhage.

PREMEDICATION

The need for sedative and vagolytic premedication as a routine before elective surgery has been hotly debated in the last decade. While accepting that a sympathetic preoperative visit, an unhurried journey to the operating room and a calm environment during induction can eliminate much of the anxiety, many patients appreciate and expect the tranquility and somnolence of sedative premedication. The need for a vagolytic can be defended before procedures which involve endobronchial instrumentation of any sort and, although the conventional doses of atropine and hyoscine do not block salivary and bronchial secretion totally, they do prevent profuse secretion interfering with manoeuvres which are sometimes technically demanding. The adverse effects of vagolytic drugs on mucociliary clearance will have worn off by the end of operation and are in any case reduced to insignificance by humidification during anaesthesia. The choice of drugs is largely a matter of individual preference and, before thoracic surgery, is rarely of critical importance. Patients scheduled for lung resection will tolerate intramuscular premedication with a morphine-based opioid combined with the sedative anticholinergic hyoscine given one to two hours before surgery. Atropine can be substituted for hyoscine in the elderly. Many anaesthetists prefer to omit opioid drugs from premedication if they intend to use epidural narcotics for postoperative analgesia, using a short-acting oral benzodiazepine such as temazepam in preference. In patients with poor lung function or upper airway obstruction, scheduled for procedures other than lung resection, it may be wise to omit premedication.

FURTHER READING

General principles of pulmonary disease

Brewis R.A.L., Gibson G.J. & Geddes D.M. (eds) (1990) *Respiratory Medicine*. Baillière, Tindall, London.
Mitchell D.M. (ed.) (1991) *Recent Advances in Respiratory Medicine*. Churchill Livingstone, London.
Seaton A., Seaton D. & Leitch A.G. (eds) (1989) *Crofton & Douglas's Respiratory Diseases*, 4th edn. Blackwell Scientific Publications, Oxford.

Radiology and related techniques

Brown K., Aberle D.R., Batra P. & Steckel R.J. (1990) Current use of imaging in the evaluation of primary mediastinal masses. *Chest*, **98**, 466–473.
Doyle P.T., Weir J., Robertson E.M., Foote A.V. & Cockburn J.S. (1986) Role of computed tomography in assessing 'operability' of bronchial carcinoma. *British Medical Journal*, **292**, 231–233.
Ell P.J., Kahn O. & Williams E.S. (1980) The management of disease and radionuclide section scanning. *British Journal of Hospital Medicine*, **24**, 225–231.
Fisher M.R. (1989) Magnetic resonance for evaluation of the thorax. *Chest*, **95**, 166–173.
Golding S. (1984) Indications for computed tomography of the chest. *Hospital Update*, **10**, 237–251.
Kerr I.H. (1974) The preoperative chest X-ray. *British Journal of Anaesthesia*, **46**, 558–563.
Underwood G.H., Hooper R.G. Axelbaum S.P. & Goodwin D.H. (1979) Computed tomographic scanning of the thorax in the staging of bronchogenic carcinoma. *New England Journal of Medicine*, **300**, 777–778.

Lung function tests and assessment of risk

Baier H. (1980) Assessment of unilateral lung function. *Anesthesiology*, **52**, 240–247.
Didolkar M.S., Moore R.H. & Takita H. (1974) Evaluation of the risk in pulmonary resection for bronchogenic carcinoma. *American Journal of Surgery* **127**, 700–703.
Hall D.R. (1974) Regional lung function after pneumonectomy. *Thorax*, **29**, 425–431.
Kristersson S. (1974) Prediction of lung function after lung surgery. A ^{133}Xe radiospirometric study of regional lung function in bronchial cancer. *Scandinavian Journal of Thoracic and Cardiovascular Surgery* (Suppl. 18).

Morgan C. (1987) Preoperative assessment of the thoracic surgical patient. In: Gothard J.W.W. (ed.) *Thoracic Anaesthesia. Clinical Anaesthesiology,* Vol. 1 pp. 1–13. Baillière, Tindall, London.

Nunn J.F., Milledge J.S., Chen D. & Dore C. (1988) Respiratory criteria of fitness for surgery and anaesthesia. *Anaesthesia,* **43**, 543–551.

Ogilvie C. (1980) Physician among surgeons: thoughts on preoperative assessment. *Thorax,* **35**, 881–883.

Olsen G.N., Block A.J., Swenson E.W., Castle J.R. & Wyune J.W. (1975) Pulmonary function evaluation of the lung resection candidate: a prospective study. *American Review of Respiratory Disease,* **111**, 379–386.

Pride N.B. (1987) The function of the lung and its investigation. In: Weatherall, D.J. Ledingham, J.G.G. & Warrell D.A. (eds) *Oxford Textbook of Medicine,* Vol. II, 2nd edn, pp. 15.25–15.35. Oxford Medical Publications, Oxford.

Tisi G.M. (1979) Preoperative evaluation of pulmonary function. Validity, indication and benefits. *American Review of Respiratory Disease,* **119**, 293–310.

Tisi G.M. (1987) Preoperative identification and evaluation of the patient with lung disease. *Medical Clinics of North America,* **71**, 399–412.

Tonnesen K.H., Dige-Peterson H., Nielsen S.L., Lauridsen, F. & Lund J.O. (1978) Lung split function test and pneumonectomy. A lower limit for operability. *Scandinavian Journal of Thoracic and Cardiovascular Surgery,* **12**, 133–136.

Exercise testing and thoracotomy

Boysen P.G., Clark C.A. & Block A.J. (1990) Graded exercise testing and post-thoracotomy complications. *Journal of Cardiothoracic Anesthesia,* **4**, 68–72.

Fishman R.S. & Systrom D.M. (1991) Preoperative cardiopulmonary exercise testing: determining the limit to exercise and predicting outcome after thoracotomy. *Journal of Cardiothoracic Anesthesia,* **5**, 614–626.

Olsen G.N. (1989) The evolving role of exercise testing prior to lung resection. *Chest,* **95**, 218–225.

Smith T.P., Kinasewitz G.T., Tucker W.Y., Spillers W.P. & George R.B. (1984) Exercise capacity as a predictor of post-thoracotomy morbidity. *American Review of Respiratory Disease,* **129**, 730–734.

Cardiac morbidity

De Bono D.P. & Rose E.L. (1991) Silent myocardial ischaemia in preoperative patients: what does it mean, and what should be done about it? *British Journal of Anaesthesia,* **67**, 307–308.

Goldman L. (1988) Assessment of the patient with known or suspected ischaemic heart disease for non-cardiac surgery. *British Journal of Anaesthesia,* **61**, 38–43.

Mangano D.T. (1990) Perioperative cardiac morbidity. *Anesthesiology,* **72**, 153–184.

Preoperative preparation

Selsby D. & Jones J.G. (1990) Some physiological and clinical aspects of chest physiotherapy. *British Journal of Anaesthesia,* **64**, 621–631.

White P.F. (1986) Pharmacological and clinical aspects of preoperative medication. *Anesthesia and Analgesia,* **65**, 963–974.

3: Diagnostic Procedures

BRONCHOSCOPY

Bronchoscopy is the most common invasive investigation required for the diagnosis of chest disease. Rigid bronchoscopy was developed in the US by Chevalier Jackson during the latter part of the 19th century and introduced slightly later to the UK by Victor Negus. The flexible, fibreoptic instrument was first described in 1968 and subsequently developed by Ikeda and colleagues.

Rigid bronchoscopy is extremely uncomfortable for a conscious subject, and although possible under local anaesthesia, is almost universally carried out using general anaesthetic techniques. Surgical opinion favours the rigid bronchoscope for the immediate preoperative location of tumours and assessment of carinal or bronchial rigidity; it is also the instrument of choice for therapeutic manoeuvres such as the extraction of foreign bodies, dilatation of strictures, or insertion of intratracheal stents (Fig. 3.1).

The fibreoptic bronchoscope is only 4–6 mm in external diameter at the tip (as compared with the 11 mm of some adult rigid bronchoscopes), is easily introduced under local anaesthesia, and can penetrate to the second or third generation of sub-segmental bronchi, including those within the right upper lobe. Small bronchial biopsies or brushings can be taken via the suction channel and this is also used for broncho-alveolar lavage and transbronchial biopsy of the lung.

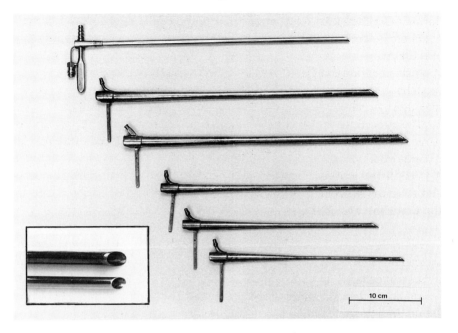

Fig. 3.1 Magill intubating bronchoscope (top) and a range of Negus bronchoscopes. *Inset.* The bevel of the Negus bronchoscope (top) is more oblique than the intubating bronchoscope and it has a rounded edge.

Bronchoscopes (from top to bottom)	Length (cm)	ID of tip (mm)
Magill intubating bronchoscope with stainless steel, parallel-sided shaft	38.2	8
Adolescent Negus bronchoscope	39.5	9
Adult Negus bronchoscope	40.0	11
Child Negus bronchoscope	30.0	8
Infant Negus bronchoscope	27.5	6
Suckling Negus bronchoscope	27.5	5

Rigid bronchoscopy

Rigid bronchoscopy is a short procedure, often lasting less than 5 minutes and rarely continuing for more than 15 minutes. Nevertheless, brevity cannot be equated with lack of risk and there are some circumstances in which the hazards are appreciable, especially if the procedure is carried out under general anaesthesia by the inexperienced. The specific problems encountered during anaesthesia for rigid bronchoscopy can be summarized as follows:

1   There is competition between bronchoscopist and anaesthetist for control of the airway.

2   Instrumentation of the upper respiratory tract is a potent cause of bronchospasm, laryngospasm, hypertension, myocardial ischaemia and cardiac dysrhythmias.

3   The procedure is sometimes indicated as an emergency on an unprepared, poorly assessed patient who already has impaired cardiovascular or respiratory function.

4   Ventilation and gas exchange can be compromised even further during and after the procedure if, for example, a lobar bronchus is obstructed by the bronchoscope, if spasm is provoked, or if haemorrhage is caused by a biopsy.

Apart from gross deformity of the mouth or neck, unequivocal contra-indications to rigid bronchoscopy, with or without general anaesthesia, are difficult to define. Conditions in which it should be avoided if possible include severe acute hypoxia, respiratory obstruction, and massive bronchopleural fistula. In some of these circumstances the hazards may be lessened by using local rather than general anaesthesia, by retaining spontaneous respiration or by using fibreoptic rather than rigid bronchoscopy. Cases in which difficulty is anticipated warrant careful assessment of the probable diagnostic or therapeutic benefit and the likely hazards, as well as a realistic appraisal of the degree of available expertise.

Anaesthetic requirements

The technique chosen must provide anaesthesia and analgesia, sufficient relaxation to allow easy passage of the rigid instrument, abolition of reflexes from the respiratory tract, and the maintenance of adequate gas exchange. Prompt recovery of consciousness, respiratory drive and the cough reflex are desirable if general anaesthesia is used, and essential after bronchial biopsy or if there are profuse secretions within the bronchial tree. It is clear from this discussion that the requirements after bronchoscopy are, to some extent, in direct conflict with those desired during the procedure. Topical analgesia, deep inhalational anaesthesia or light anaesthesia with an intravenous agent and muscle relaxant all fulfil at least some of these requirements. Deep inhalational anaesthesia is almost never used now unless there is both a specific indication for preserving spontaneous ventilation and general anaesthesia is also considered necessary, e.g. some instances of respiratory obstruction. In general, local anaesthetic techniques are reserved for fibre-optic bronchoscopy.

Topical analgesia

The procedure is explained to the patient who is then given an amethocaine lozenge to suck and advised that the solution resulting from it should be dispersed throughout the mouth and then swallowed to ensure anaesthesia of the lips, tongue and pharynx. It is essential that this be done before any premedication with a vagolytic is given so that salivary secretion is preserved. Instrumentation within the mouth and tracheobronchial tree is a potent stimulus to local secretion and it is customary to complete premedication with intramuscular atropine and a light sedative if desired.

The rest of the local anaesthetic is given once the patient is in the endoscopy room. The superior laryngeal nerves are anaesthetized by applying swabs soaked in 4% lignocaine to the pyriform fossae and then the trachea is anaesthetized by injecting lignocaine over the back of the tongue. Alternatively, the glottis and vocal cords can be anaesthetized via an intratracheal injection of lignocaine, or more simply by spraying lignocaine on to the vocal cords directly, via the suction channel of the fibreoptic bronchoscope, as the instrument is advanced. The total dose of plain lignocaine used should be monitored carefully with regard to the size and physical status of the patient, bearing in mind that the drug will be rapidly absorbed systemically. The patient is ready for bronchoscopy a few minutes later when the effect of the local anaesthetic will be at its maximum and any coughing caused by its introduction will have ceased. If endotracheal intubation is planned via the fibreoptic bronchoscope it is useful to treat the nasal mucosa with cotton buds soaked in 10% cocaine solution to provide both anaesthesia and vasoconstriction.

Additional sedation, in the form of intravenous midazolam or diazepam, may be required during the procedure. Hypoxaemia occurs during instrumentation of the airway under local anaesthesia, particularly when combined with sedation. Monitoring should include non-invasive blood pressure measurement, electrocardiogram (ECG) and pulse oximetry.

Inhalational anaesthesia

The subject is premedicated lightly, often with only intramuscular atropine. The choice of inhalational agent will depend on personal preference and halothane, isoflurane or ethrane can be used. The author still finds halothane the easiest agent to use in these circumstances, although the risk of hepatitis and sensitization of the myocardium to raised arterial carbon dioxide levels must be borne in mind. The depth of halothane anaesthesia changes rapidly so that a patient anaesthetized to the point of respiratory arrest can lighten to an unacceptable degree during all but the shortest procedure. As a result, bronchoscopy and the administration of more anaesthetic have to alternate and the bronchoscopist is at risk of sedation from exhaled halothane. Fortunately, inhalational anaesthesia is often only indicated for induction and intravenous anaesthesia can be instituted once the airway has been secured, or more commonly once the mobility of the vocal cords has been assessed.

Intravenous anaesthesia

This is the usual choice for bronchoscopy under general anaesthesia, and is based on light narcosis and total paralysis with gas exchange supported or controlled by one of three techniques: a ventilating bronchoscope, 'jet ventilation' utilizing the Venturi principle, or high frequency jet ventilation (HFJV).

'Traditional' premedication with papaveretum and hyoscine or atropine is often prescribed but this choice highlights the conflicting requirements of conditions during and immediately after bronchoscopy. A more logical alternative to papaveretum is a benzodiazepine as an anxiolytic and amnesic agent, although the action of some of these drugs is unduly prolonged. The conventional intramuscular doses of both hyoscine and atropine are insufficient to suppress vagal reflexes entirely and intravenous atropine given as required during the procedure is, theoretically, a preferable choice. Atropine is preferable to hyoscine to prevent prolonged sedation but glycopyrrolate may ultimately prove the most successful vagolytic.

Induction can be carried out with any suitable induction agent such as etomidate, thiopentone or propofol. The short-acting agent propofol is eminently suitable for use during bronchoscopy. It has been shown to attenuate the haemodynamic responses to bronchoscopy (an increase in heart rate and both systemic and pulmonary hypertension) without the need for pretreatment with alfentanil. Propofol can, providing hypotension does not occur, be given in generous doses to prevent awareness during bronchoscopy. For particularly long procedures an infusion of propofol can also be used to provide anaesthesia (Table 3.1) and yet, because of the drug's rapid elimination, this will still allow rapid awakening of the patient when desired.

Suxamethonium is given after induction for an isolated bronchoscopy. The anaesthetist then inflates the lungs with oxygen and in some instances may spray the vocal cords with lignocaine in order to attenuate the response to laryngeal intubation and to minimize the possibility of postoperative laryngospasm. The evidence that lignocaine prevents laryngospasm is,

Chapter 3

Table 3.1 Induction and maintenance of propofol anaesthesia. This regime, taken from Roberts *et al.* (1988), achieved a mean propofol blood level greater than 3 μg/ml, with a satisfactory level of anaesthesia

---

Induction
1 mg/kg propofol

Maintenance
Propofol
   10 mg/kg/h for 10 minutes
   8 mg/kg/h for 8 minutes
   6 mg/kg/h continuously thereafter

---

however, tenuous, particularly if the procedure is prolonged. The lungs are inflated again with oxygen for a few breaths just before insertion of the bronchoscope and, once this is within the trachea, the selected method of ventilation is instituted. Anaesthesia and muscular relaxation are maintained by increments of the induction agent and suxamethonium, although it is notoriously difficult to judge the depth of anaesthesia accurately. If the bronchoscopy is undertaken prior to a longer procedure such as mediasti-notomy or thoracotomy a non-depolarizing muscle relaxant such as atracu-rium or vecuronium can be used from the outset, provided there are no contraindications such as the likelihood of a difficult intubation. Once the bronchoscope has been withdrawn, at the end of the procedure, the patient is turned on his or her side with the biopsied or diseased side downwards to avoid soiling the contralateral lung with blood or secretions. Spontaneous ventilation is re-established while oxygen is administered through a facemask and the patient should remain under immediate observation until there is no anxiety at all about the adequacy of protective reflexes. Nothing should be given by mouth for 3 hours afterwards if lignocaine has been used.

Monitoring

Non-invasive blood pressure measurement, an ECG and pulse oximetry are mandatory during rigid bronchoscopy.

Ventilation during rigid bronchoscopy

Methods of ventilation currently used during rigid bronchoscopy include the ventilating bronchoscope, Venturi ventilation and HFJV. Apnoeic ventilation, using oxygen insufflation via a fine catheter, has largely been abandoned because of the progressive rise in arterial carbon dioxide tension associated with this technique.

Ventilating bronchoscope. Modern bronchoscopes of the Storz type can be used as ventilating instruments. A side arm allows ventilation via an anaesthetic circuit and the proximal end of the scope is sealed with a sliding glass window or a rubber diaphragm to allow passage of an optical telescope. Small paediatric Storz bronchoscopes are particularly suitable for use as ventilating bronchoscopes (Figs 3.2 and 3.3). An instrument of appropriate size is likely to provide an adequate fit in a child's trachea (which is relatively narrower than the larynx) and ventilation can be achieved manually via a T-piece circuit even when an optical telescope is placed down the bronchoscope. A child can, therefore, be kept anaesthetized during bronchoscopy with an easily eliminated and safe inhalational agent. Venturi ventilation, which does not provide a route for anaesthesia and is more risky in the narrow paediatric airway, can largely be avoided in children.

Venturi ventilation. Sanders first described 'injector' techniques of ventilation based on the Venturi entrainment principle in 1967. This remains the most common form of ventilation during rigid bronchoscopy. Oxygen from a high pressure source is injected intermittently through a narrow needle placed at the proximal end of the bronchoscope (Figs 3.4 and 3.5). The Venturi effect

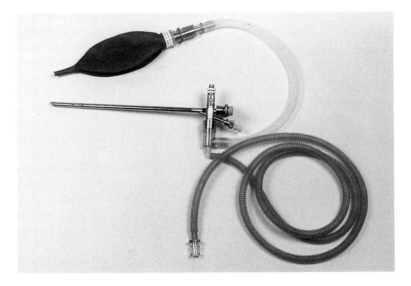

Fig. 3.2 A paediatric ventilating bronchoscope (Storz) with T-piece circuit attached.

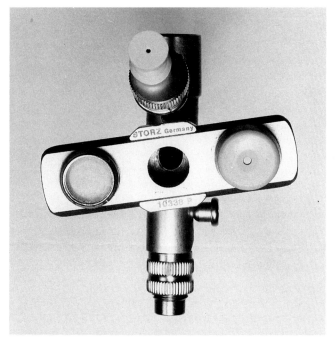

Fig. 3.3 Close up view of slide arrangement at proximal end of ventilating bronchoscope. A glass window or rubber diaphragm (for telescope) can occlude the end of the scope or alternatively it can be left open for instrumentation.

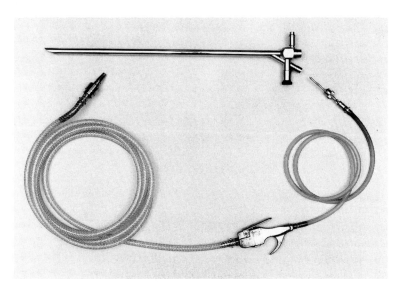

Fig. 3.4 Storz bronchoscope and injector.

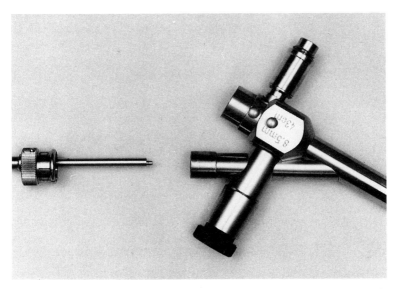

Fig. 3.5 Proximal end of the Storz bronchoscope and detail of the needle used to provide ventilation by the injector technique. Note the appropriate size of needle (16 gauge) just protruding from the tip of a larger needle.

which this creates entrains atmospheric air so that the lungs can be inflated with oxygen-enriched air as long as the distal end of the bronchoscope is beyond the larynx. Expiration occurs passively through and around the bronchoscope. The endoscopist has an unhindered view with good access for instrumentation, and the 'blow-back' of gases from the proximal end of the bronchoscope is usually considered tolerable, particularly if protective spectacles are worn. The system consists of a high pressure source of oxygen (usually pipeline pressure at 410 kPa; approximately 60 psi), an on/off tap, high pressure connecting tubing and a needle of suitable size. Several systems have been described which use a modified ventilator to supply the driving gas, but these seem unnecessarily complex for use during what is usually a short procedure.

It is essential that the size of the needle should match that of the bronchoscope so that good air entrainment is achieved without creating excessive airway pressure. A 16 standard wire gauge (SWG) needle coupled to a driving gas pressure of 410 kPa is usually used with an adult Negus or Storz bronchoscope and gives a maximum inflation pressure of 25–30 cmH$_2$O (2.5–3.0 kPa) with a peak gas flow of 170 litres/min at the distal end. A needle of similar size in a suckling (small paediatric) bronchoscope would produce pressures over 100 cmH$_2$O (10 kPa), but a 19 gauge needle in the same bronchoscope would limit this to approximately 15 cmH$_2$O (1.5 kPa). Typical maximum pressures achieved with various sizes of needle and bronchoscope are summarized in Table 3.2.

The extent of air entrainment and the pressure created can be altered if the driving gas pressure is adjusted with a reducing valve attached to an oxygen cylinder. However, the system is safer if the driving gas pressure remains constant and appropriately-sized injector needles are used for standard sizes of bronchoscope. Should there be any doubt about the maximum pressure created by any system, it is a simple matter to place the bronchoscope, with its side-holes occluded, into a measuring cylinder filled with water and note the depth at which bubbles just begin to appear when the injector is operated.

Another cause of excessive pressure is obstruction of the proximal end of the bronchoscope when it is also a tight fit at the larynx or elsewhere within the tracheobronchial tree. This is uncommon in adults, even when telescopes and biopsy forceps are in use, but is a greater risk during instrumentation through a paediatric bronchoscope (see section on damage to the lungs and airways on p. 40). A final factor which must be considered is the impedance to inflation of the patient's lungs and airways. Increasing impedance results in less air entrainment, a smaller tidal volume but an increased oxygen concentration. A standard device is occasionally inadequate for patients with high airway resistance or poor pulmonary compliance, in which case a larger needle can be used to generate a higher inflation pressure.

High frequency jet ventilation (HFJV). HFJV, at rates between 60 up to several hundred times/min, was developed in Sweden to provide adequate alveolar ventilation at a low airway pressure. This method of ventilation has not been widely adopted for routine bronchoscopy but has been used for more difficult airway procedures such as the insertion of intratracheal stents and resection of tracheal stenosis. HFJV can also be used to provide ventilation, via an endotracheal tube with a built-in 'jetting' port, when general anaesthesia is employed for fibreoptic bronchoscopy.

Complications of rigid bronchoscopy

Interference with respiration is undoubtedly the most serious hazard, usually caused either by obstruction, or drug-induced depression of central drive or muscle tone. It is equally important to realize that these risks are often greatest after rather than during the examination and, if there is any doubt about the adequacy of spontaneous ventilation or the patency of the airway,

Table 3.2 Maximum inflation pressure achieved with various Venturi bronchoscope injector systems (driving pressure 410 kPa)

Negus bronchoscope	Injector needle		Typical max. pressure[†]	
	Size* SWG	Internal diameter (mm)	cmH$_2$O	kPa
Adult	14	1.20	50	4.9
Adult	16	1.20	25–30	2.45–2.94
Adult	17	1.10	23–25	2.26–2.45
Child	19	0.69	14–18	1.37–1.77
Suckling	19	0.69	15	1.47

* Needle sizes are expressed as SWG but some commercially available needles do not conform exactly to British standards. The internal diameters shown here are from the injector range manufactured by Penlon Ltd, Abingdon
† The use of entrainment needles in bronchoscopes does not produce a 'pure' Venturi by engineering standards and entrainment will vary to some extent on the design of the bronchoscope, the length of the needle and the manufacturing tolerance of any bend that has been incorporated in the design

it is safer to pass an endotracheal tube and continue positive pressure ventilation until the anxiety has passed, than to adopt a policy of 'wait and see'.

A particular circumstance which warrants special consideration is haemorrhage caused by biopsy of a friable tumour or, worse still, an over-deep biopsy which has penetrated a major vessel. If there is significant bleeding at the end of the procedure, it is safer to leave the bronchoscope in place so that suction can be continued under direct vision until the patient is awake and has adequate reflexes. Gross haemorrhage is uncommon but can sometimes be controlled by inserting a blocker (see Chapter 5) to isolate the source of bleeding and apply pressure to it. This approach works well in expert hands if the source of the bleeding is superficial. An alternative, often more readily available, is to pass a double-lumen tube so that ventilation can be secured through the non-involved lung while posture and suction are used to drain blood from the site of biopsy.

Adverse reactions to anaesthetic drugs are infrequent and only the use of lignocaine need be considered critically. As previously stated it is important to avoid exceeding the maximum recommended dose (3 mg/kg), particularly when it is used as the sole agent, and either the volume or strength of the solution should be adjusted for small or debilitated patients. Lignocaine is absorbed very readily from the respiratory tract but lower blood levels have been reported when parts of the larynx are sprayed separately than when a single bolus is delivered between the cords.

The use of lignocaine during bronchoscopy under general anaesthesia is more controversial. In theory, topical analgesia allows a lighter plane of general anaesthesia and hence quicker awakening, as well as some protection against bronchospasm or laryngospasm induced by instrumentation. However, continued depression of the cough reflex is undesirable after bronchoscopy and, although topical lignocaine may reduce the incidence or severity of laryngospasm after short procedures, this does not appear to be so if bronchoscopy is prolonged.

Dysrhythmias can be provoked by hypoxia, hypercarbia, instrumentation of the larynx and trachea, or by incremental doses of suxamethonium. The efficiency of the technique of ventilation is an important determinant, clearly demonstrated by a reported incidence of rhythm disturbances ranging from 44% during apnoeic oxygenation to 14% with a ventilating bronchoscope and only 4% with a Venturi injector.

Bradycardia related to incremental doses of suxamethonium should be treated with intravenous atropine. Other dysrhythmias usually respond to simple measures such as improved ventilation, deepening the level of anaesthesia, or movement of the bronchoscope; specific drug therapy is rarely required.

Damage to the lungs or airways is a rare but serious complication of any technique which can allow a high pressure to build up beyond the tip of the bronchoscope. This can only occur if gas cannot escape either through the bronchoscope or around it, a situation which exists when the lumen is occluded, usually with a telescope, and the bronchoscope fits snugly at or beyond the larynx. Jet ventilation used without due consideration for the relative size of the instrument and the injector is a potent cause of excessive pressure, but an insufflation catheter and bronchoscope between them may completely occupy a narrow trachea and so create similar conditions. Pneumomediastinum, surgical emphysema, lung rupture, pneumothorax and air embolism can all result and a number of fatalities have been recorded.

Awareness during bronchoscopy under general anaesthesia is disturbingly common when the modern technique of light intravenous anaesthesia and muscular relaxation is sued. The reported incidence varies from 1 to 4% and includes accounts of instrumentation, paralysis, conversation (often the most distressing) or of chest pain. It is worth warning patients preoperatively that they may recollect withdrawal of the bronchoscope and suction in the mouth and throat because it is important for them to wake quickly so that they can breathe and cough well. However, this is scant comfort for the patient who remembers the entire procedure.

Premedication with specific anxiolytic or amnesic drugs is more likely to prevent recall than papaveretum, even when combined with hyoscine, but the effect is dose-dependent and consequently the duration of action is prolonged to an unacceptable degree. A rigid regime for the use of intravenous induction agents is superior to one relying on clinical judgment and, in one report, recall was eliminated when methohexitone was given in an initial dose of 1.5 mg/kg, followed by 25% of this dose every 2 minutes. The use of propofol by infusion is also likely to reduce the incidence of awareness during bronchoscopy particularly if given by a strict protocol. Mixtures of nitrous oxide and oxygen have been delivered through an insufflating catheter or ventilating bronchoscope and have been recommended as the driving gas for a Venturi system. However, even 70% nitrous oxide in these circumstances does not result in a blood level high enough to alter the incidence of awareness; this remains a common problem and one which has not been resolved completely.

Rigid bronchoscopy for endobronchial laser therapy and diathermy resection

Surgical lasers are used to resect tracheobronchial tumours. This surgery is of a palliative nature often carried out in elderly and debilitated patients in order to relieve severe bronchial or even tracheal obstruction. The laser is used to resect and cauterize intraluminal tumours in order to relieve breathlessness and haemoptysis. Endobronchial laser therapy can be carried out under local anaesthesia combined with sedation. Recent experience, however, suggests that general anaesthesia provides superior operating conditions so that palliation can be achieved with fewer treatment sessions and without the problem of bleeding and asphyxiation that has led to death in series where local anaesthesia has been employed.

A number of different lasers have been used for endobronchial surgery including the carbon dioxide and neodymium yttrium–aluminium–garnet (Nd YAG) lasers. The thermal effect of lasers is the main basis for their efficacy but this also has significant implications for their use during general anaesthesia. There is a significant fire hazard when lasers are used in the presence of conventional endotracheal tubes, particularly if the inspired oxygen concentration is high. Foil wrapped, or even metal, endotracheal tubes have been utilized during laser treatment but a simpler approach is to use a metal, rigid bronchoscope. Following induction of anaesthesia a rigid adult bronchoscope is introduced into the airway and Venturi ventilation commenced (see above). A fibreoptic bronchoscope is then passed down the rigid instrument to reach the area of tumour. Ventilation is continued and an optical fibre is introduced down the biopsy channel of the fibreoptic instrument in order to transmit the laser beam to the required site. The laser is used to resect tumour and both biopsy forceps and suction catheters can be passed intermittently down the rigid bronchoscope to remove blood and tumour debris. At times it will be necessary to suspend Venturi ventilation whilst smoke particles are suctioned from the airway. This does not present an unreasonable hazard with appropriate monitoring.

Anaesthesia for laser therapy is carried out on the lines previously described for prolonged bronchoscopy, paralysis being achieved with atracurium or vecuronium and anaesthesia maintained with propofol. Induction of anaesthesia is particularly hazardous in the presence of upper airway obstruction and its severity should be assessed preoperatively both clinically and from the chest X-ray and computerized tomography (CT) scan. The theoretical advantages of an inhalational induction are rarely applicable to this type of palliative surgery carried out in elderly debilitated patients and may only be considered in extreme circumstances. After preoxygenation anaesthesia is induced slowly with an intravenous agent. This is followed by intravenous suxamethonium (rather than a non-depolarizing agent) if there is any doubt about the airway. A skilled bronchoscopist should be present from the outset. Once the airway has been secured and ventilation established via the rigid bronchoscope, atracurium or vecuronium can be administered.

At the end of laser bronchoscopy, which may be a prolonged procedure, most patients can be extubated and allowed to breathe spontaneously. A number of patients will, however, require a period of postoperative mechanical ventilation. This requirement relates to a variety of factors including existing muscular weakness, inadequate reversal of muscle relaxants and significant stridor.

Diathermy resection is an alternative and somewhat simpler treatment mode for the resection of endobronchial tumours. A diathermy resection device, with an incorporated telescope, is used to remove tumour under direct vision via a rigid bronchoscope. Ventilation is achieved via a Venturi device and the anaesthetic considerations are similar to those discussed for laser therapy.

Rigid bronchoscopy for tracheobronchial stent insertion

This is discussed in Chapter 9.

Fibreoptic bronchoscopy

The fibreoptic bronchoscope is usually passed through the nose under local anaesthesia. Premedication with a light sedative is customary, possibly combined with a vagolytic agent. The larynx, trachea and bronchi are anaesthetized under direct vision by injecting lignocaine through the suction channel of the bronchoscope as it is advanced (Fig. 3.6). Many anaesthetists, however, prefer a more rigid and systematic approach to topical anaesthesia of the respiratory tract (as described above), particularly if endotracheal intubation is planned via this route.

Complications of the procedure are infrequent and rarely serious. Hypoxaemia is common while the bronchoscope is within the bronchial tree and should be treated with supplemental oxygen. Bronchospasm may occur during the procedure but severe spasm and laryngospasm are surprisingly rare. Troublesome haemorrhage is an occasional problem after bronchial or transbronchial biopsy and is more difficult to control than during rigid bronchoscopy because of the narrow lumen of the suction channel. Pneumothorax after transbronchial biopsy is uncommon if the procedure is carried out under radiological control.

General anaesthesia for fibreoptic bronchoscopy

Fibreoptic bronchoscopy is sometimes carried out electively under general anaesthesia, even in adults, and it may be required for diagnosis or treatment in the intensive care unit. It is a simple matter to pass the fibreoptic bronchoscope (external diameter 6 mm) through an 8 mm or 9 mm endotracheal tube; ventilation can be continued without difficulty, preferably by hand, provided the bronchoscope is inserted through a diaphragm which seals the endotracheal tube connector (Fig. 3.7). The annulus between the bronchoscope and the endotracheal tube should be sufficient to allow free passage of gas in and out of the lungs as well as easy movement of the bronchoscope within the tube. The introduction of ultra-thin paediatric bronchoscopes allows a similar technique to be used in children. Anaesthesia can conveniently be maintained with an inhalational agent or, alternatively, a propofol infusion in adults. Paralysis is achieved with suxamethonium for a very short bronchoscopy or either atracurium or vecuronium for a longer procedure.

HFJV can also be used to provide ventilation during fibreoptic bronchoscopy, either via an endotracheal tube or a catheter placed through the vocal cords. Jet ventilation (or the use of the Sanders injector) must be used with extreme caution in these latter circumstances. Expiration occurs passively

Chapter 3

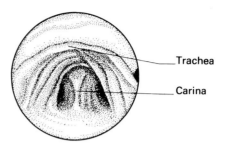

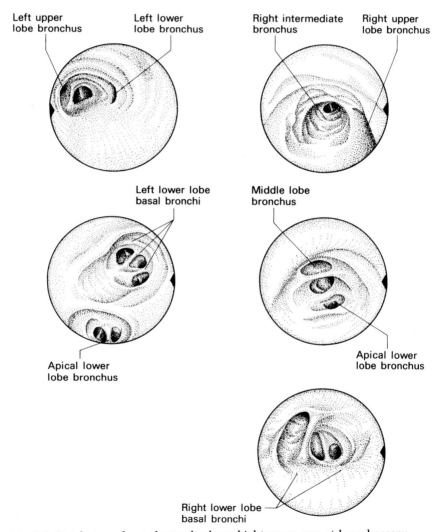

Fig. 3.6 Serial views down the tracheobronchial tree as seen at bronchoscopy.

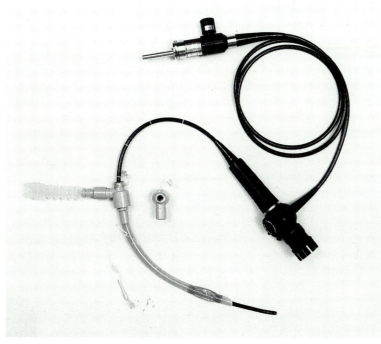

Fig. 3.7 Fibreoptic bronchoscope passed through an endotracheal tube. It has been introduced through a self-sealing Portex connector which is also shown separately.

around the outside of the catheter and any obstruction, even closure of the vocal cords, will allow a dangerously high pressure to build up quickly. A comparable hazard exists if the catheter is pushed on and impacts in a bronchus or is jammed against the wall of the trachea. The delivery of gas at high pressure under these conditions makes pneumothorax and fatal air embolism very probable. Pressure monitoring devices and pressure limiting valves have been advocated to minimize these risks. It is also essential to ensure that the vocal cords remain totally paralysed throughout the procedure, that inspiration is short by comparison with expiration, and that hyperinflation of the chest and distension of the neck veins are never allowed to occur.

BRONCHOGRAPHY

Bronchography, a method of delineating the bronchial tree with radio-opaque contrast medium, was first carried out in 1922. It is used mainly for the diagnosis and evaluation of bronchiectasis and hence its value is declining in developed countries because of a lower incidence of the antecedent conditions — measles, whooping cough and primary tuberculosis — and the more widespread use of antibiotics in these and other childhood infections. CT scanning is now also used to evaluate bronchiectasis and therefore bronchography is carried out infrequently in the UK.

Bronchography can be carried out using local anaesthesia combined with a sedative technique whilst the contrast medium is delivered to specific lobes via a fibreoptic bronchoscope. Occasionally general anaesthesia is indicated.

Contrast materials and technical aspects

Up until recently the iodine-containing radio-opaque substance Dionosil (propyliodine BP) has been the agent of choice for bronchography. This contrast medium is no longer manufactured, although large stocks remain. In the future, if bronchography is still indicated, a suitable replacement substance must be found.

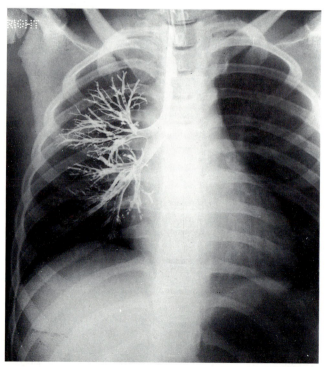

Fig. 3.8 Postero-anterior view of a normal bronchogram obtained in a young child under general anaesthesia.

Water-based Dionosil is currently used for bronchography at the author's base hospital because it produces satisfactory bronchograms (Figs 3.8–3.10) and is rapidly cleared from the tracheobronchial tree. The water-based compound is very irritant, however, and has been said to cause pneumonitis. Dionosil in its oily form is, surprisingly, less irritant and is therefore preferred in some centres. It does, however, take 2–3 days to be completely cleared from the lungs. Sensitivity reactions can occur with Dionosil, even though it is a relatively inert iodine-containing compound, and are usually manifest at an acute asthmatic response. Skin tests for iodine sensitivity are unreliable and, if hypersensitivity is suspected, corticosteroids should be given before the examination or an alternative contrast material such as barium carboxymethyl cellulose can be used.

Hypoxia and some degree of obstruction to the small airways are inevitable during bronchography and pulse oximetry is mandatory during the procedure. Bronchography is particularly hazardous in infants under 1 year and should be avoided in this age group if at all possible or, if regarded as essential, confined to one lung only and the dose of contrast medium kept to

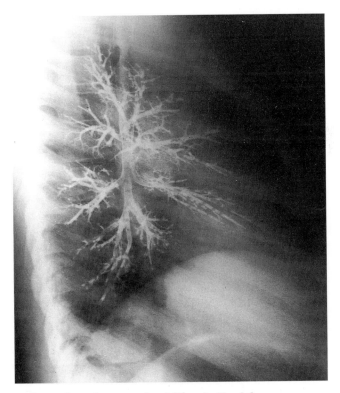

Fig. 3.9 Lateral view bronchogram of a child as in Fig. 3.8.

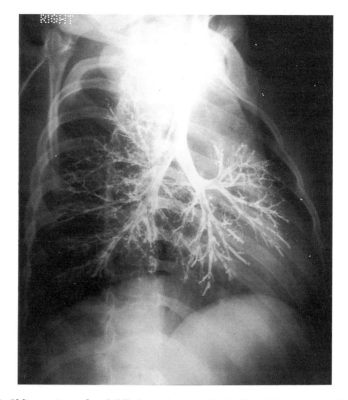

Fig. 3.10 Oblique view of a child's bronchogram (as in Figs 3.8 and 3.9). There is trifurcation of the left upper lobe.

a minimum. In adults, 20–25 ml Dionosil is usually sufficient for each lung but up to 30 ml can be instilled on each side if necessary in a pathological lung. In children, 0.75–1.0 ml of contrast medium per year of age is considered to be an appropriate dose.

The right side is studied first when both lungs are to be examined during one procedure because a lateral view is needed to demonstrate the bronchial anatomy on this side and this will be confused if there is residual contrast material on the left side. A tilting table with cradle should be used if possible so that the patient can be positioned easily and X-rays exposed without further disturbance. Fluoroscopic control during injection is desirable and postero-anterior, right oblique and right lateral films are taken when optimum filling has been achieved. The left lung can then be studied adequately with an oblique view so that contrast material in the right lung does not interfere with interpretation.

General anaesthesia for bronchography

Children and unusually nervous or uncooperative adults require general anaesthesia for bronchography and this presents several problems. Respiratory function is usually compromised already, most patients are expectorating considerable quantities of sputum in spite of preoperative preparation, and the introduction of contrast material interferes with respiratory function even further. As with bronchoscopy, the requirements during and after the procedure are in conflict, with a need for abolition of the cough reflex during the examination, but an equally cogent need for the rapid return of reflexes afterwards so that sputum and contrast material can be expelled from the proximal parts of the bronchial tree.

Preoperative preparation

The patient. The indication for bronchography will be clear at the preoperative visit. If the patient suffers from bronchiectasis, it is important to discover the extent of interference with respiratory function, whether or not there is a tendency to airway obstruction and, if so, whether this is labile, the volume of sputum produced each day, its quality and whether it has been cleared as completely as possible by postural drainage and antibiotics. It is also useful to know if haemoptysis is a frequent feature of the disease process.

Conventional premedication with an oral sedative such as temazepam is usually satisfactory. An anti-sialogogue is not mandatory.

The equipment. All anaesthetic equipment should be checked with particular care. A non-radio-opaque warming blanket is useful when small children are anaesthetized and a torch or small light should be available. All drugs which may be used for anaesthesia or resuscitation should be prepared in advance. It is useful to draw up the maximum, on the basis of weight or surface area, of drugs such as suxamethonium so that oversedation or prolonged paralysis can be avoided. Syringes should be clearly marked with large letters or, preferably, syringes of different sizes should be used for the different agents, diluting the drugs as necessary. An endotracheal tube of suitable size for the patient is chosen and a nasogastric tube is cut to protrude approximately 1–2 cm from the distal end of the former.

Anaesthetic technique

Monitoring consisting of an ECG, non-invasive blood pressure measurement and pulse oximetry is instituted prior to anaesthesia. Induction with intra-venous propofol (or an inhalational agent in children) is followed by intravenous suxamethonium and endotracheal intubation. An inhalational agent, such as isoflurane, can be used to maintain anaesthesia in an air/oxygen mixture. The use of 100% oxygen or oxygen in nitrous oxide may promote lobar collapse if the bronchi are totally blocked by contrast material.

Instillation of contrast material

Manual ventilation is used to control respiration and intermittent suxame-thonium is administered when apnoea is required. The nasogastric tube is advanced just beyond the tip of the endotracheal tube (via a seal in the tube connector or more simply through the open end of the tube). Then, with the patient appropriately positioned, and temporarily apnoeic, the contrast medium is slowly injected down the nasogastric tube and into the airway. The lungs are screened radiographically and gentle manual inflation em-ployed to outline the bronchi of interest with contrast medium. A permanent X-ray record is taken. As much contrast material as possible is removed by suction once one lung has been studied and prior to studying the second side.

The anaesthetic is terminated as soon as satisfactory films have been obtained. Suction and physiotherapy are used to remove as much contrast material as possible from the respiratory tract but often very little is obtained. The endotracheal tube should remain in place until there is an active cough reflex and the patient should be nursed flat or head-down but with the healthier of the two lungs uppermost. Humidified oxygen should be given during the recovery period; gentle percussion of the chest and encourage-ment to cough are useful in helping to clear both bronchial secretions and residual contrast material. Laryngospasm is an occasional complication, particularly in infants, and resuscitation equipment should be readily available.

MEDIASTINOSCOPY AND MEDIASTINOTOMY

Carlens used mediastinoscopy to explore the potential space on both sides of the superior mediastinum through a small cervical incision, and reported his experience in 1959. The procedure allows inspection and biopsy under direct vision of paratracheal, superior tracheobronchial and anterior parts of the subcarinal lymph nodes (Fig. 3.11). However, tumours of the thymus and anterior mediastinum are inaccessible because they lie in front of the great vessels and can only be approached through an anterior mediastinotomy.

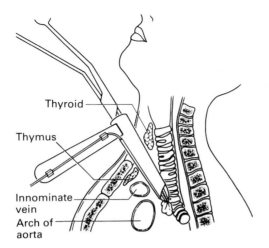

Fig. 3.11 Mediastinoscopy.

The procedure is of value in two circumstances: as a means of establishing a histological diagnosis when mediastinal lymphadenopathy is known to be present but is of uncertain aetiology, and as part of the preoperative assessment of patients with potentially operable carcinoma of the bronchus. The superior mediastinum is difficult to explore radiologically but, if disease is known to be present in it, thoracotomy and attempted resection for bronchial carcinoma are usually regarded as inadvisable. CT scanning, as discussed in Chapter 2, has decreased the need for mediastinoscopy in the staging of lung cancer. If the mediastinum is clear on CT scanning, and there is no other evidence of secondary spread, thoracotomy can be undertaken without a preliminary staging procedure. When enlarged nodes are present in the mediastinum on CT scanning mediastinoscopy or left anterior mediastinotomy is indicated. This is because it is currently impossible to differentiate, with the available scanning techniques, whether a node is enlarged as a result of secondary tumour spread or simply as a consequence of reactive hyperplasia.

Surgical aspects

A small incision is made above the supra-sternal notch and the pretracheal muscles are separated by blunt dissection until the pretracheal fascia can be incised. Blunt dissection is continued along the anterior surface of the trachea until it is possible to slide the mediastinoscope into position (Fig. 3.11). Any structure which is to be biopsied should be aspirated first with a fine needle to ensure it is not vascular. Haemorrhage can still be a problem and small vessels are sealed using an insulated diathermy point mounted in a fine sucker. More serious bleeding can usually be controlled by packing the mediastinum with swabs, but severe haemorrhage cannot always be stopped in this way and usually indicates damage to a large vessel which can only be secured by proceeding to immediate thoracotomy. Other complications include pneumothorax, haemothorax, air embolism, paralysis of either or both recurrent laryngeal nerves, and hemiplegia caused by damage to the innominate artery. Deaths related to anaesthesia have contributed as much as 50% of the mortality in some series, and neither the anaesthetic nor the procedure should be delegated to the inexperienced. In experienced hands, however, the procedure should be very safe.

Anaesthesia for mediastinoscopy

Preoperative assessment

Mediastinoscopy is most hazardous in the presence of superior vena caval obstruction or obstruction to the upper airway. Both may worsen as a result of endotracheal anaesthesia, and further deterioration will occur post-operatively if there is significant bleeding within the mediastinum or if coughing and straining are features of the recovery period. Superior caval obstruction is most dangerous when it develops acutely because collateral vessels will not be present, but the converse is true of respiratory obstruction because rapidly worsening symptoms often indicate that oedema or a rapidly expanding but soft mass are responsible, rather than a rigid obstruction. Some indication of the site, severity and nature of respiratory obstruction can often be obtained from CT scans and X-rays of the thoracic inlet.

These hazards must be considered for each patient against the possible therapeutic benefit which may result if a positive diagnosis can be established. Patients without these two conditions are assessed preoperatively in the usual way but it is worth noting that coagulation disorders or the neuromyopathic complications of some types of bronchial carcinoma may be relevant in individual cases (see Chapter 10).

Anaesthetic management

There are few constraints on premedication unless signs of caval or tracheal obstruction are present. Then sedative premedication should be kept to a minimum to avoid respiratory depression and prevent worsening obstruction as a result of any diminution in muscle tone.

Oral intubation with a non-kinking endotracheal tube follows an intravenous induction and short-acting muscle relaxant in the majority of cases. Preoxygenation is essential for those with either upper airway or superior caval obstruction, but the theoretical attractions of an inhalational induction are not borne out in practice because straining and coughing or respiratory depression aggravate venous engorgement, and spontaneous respiration may cease before a sufficient depth of anaesthesia is reached to allow laryngoscopy. This is likely to be difficult anyway, particularly in those with caval obstruction, and smooth atraumatic intubation is most likely to be achieved by creating optimum conditions. Orotracheal intubation is virtually always possible, even though the trachea is displaced or distorted, but it is wise to have a range of small endotracheal tubes available when tracheal narrowing is known to be present.

The procedure is carried out with the patient supine. The neck is extended by placing a sandbag under the shoulders, and the head is supported on a ring to prevent overextension of the neck and allow the face to be turned slightly away from the side which is to be explored. A head-up tilt minimizes venous engorgement but the risks of hypotension and air embolism must be remembered if this is more than minimal.

Controlled ventilation with an inhalational agent such as isoflurane in an air/oxygen mixture prevents coughing and straining and avoids deep inhalational anaesthesia. The procedure is rarely prolonged and so the dose and type of muscle relaxant should be chosen with this in mind; either atracurium or vecuronium is usually appropriate. The ECG should be recorded throughout and the blood pressure measured non-invasively on the left arm because unreliable values will be detected on the right if the innominate artery is compressed. Pulse oximetry is mandatory. An intravenous infusion through a large-bore cannula should be established in every case but cannulation of central veins is unnecessary and, indeed, should be avoided in those with caval obstruction. At the end of the procedure, particular attention should be given to the adequacy of reversal of muscle relaxants and to the ability of the patient to maintain a clear airway after extubation.

Anterior mediastinotomy

Exploration of the anterior mediastinum through the bed of the second costal cartilage allows access to tumours and lymph nodes which would be inaccessible by mediastinoscopy and also provides a convenient route for open lung biopsy. The incision is larger and more obtrusive than that used for mediastinoscopy, but the incidence of complications is lower because structures can be visualized and controlled more readily. The pleural cavity is not opened intentionally, unless lung biopsy is also indicated, but inadvertent entry is common especially on the right. If the pleura is opened this is drained during surgical closure. A wide-bore nasogastric tube is placed in the mediastinotomy wound and the lung is re-expanded by the anaesthetist. As the muscle suture line is near completion a sustained inflation pressure is applied to the lung whilst the tube is withdrawn and the suture line is completed by the surgeon to prevent re-occurrence of the pneumothorax.

The anaesthetic considerations for mediastinotomy are very similar to those for mediastinoscopy except that the position of the head is unimportant and the blood pressure can be measured on either arm because there is little chance of compression of the innominate artery. Some surgeons actually excise a portion of the second costal cartilage and if this is carried out opioid supplements such as fentanyl or alfentanil should be given.

THORACOSCOPY

Thoracoscopy allows direct inspection and biopsy of the pleura through a small incision in the chest wall. It was often carried out in the early days of thoracic surgery to divide pleural adhesions which prevented therapeutic collapse of a tuberculous lung when an artificial pneumothorax had been induced. Diagnostic thoracoscopy has remained in use ever since and is currently the subject of renewed interest.

Thoracoscopy is a useful method of investigating pleural disease and persistent pleural effusions when biopsy and aspiration are negative. There is also increasing interest in the therapeutic application of thoracoscopy for a variety of procedures including the insufflation of talc to create a pleurodesis, transthoracic vagotomy and even endoscopic pleurectomy! A specially designed thoracoscope is available commercially (Storz) but a laparoscope is a suitable alternative. A small light on a malleable probe can be used to improve illumination in inaccessible corners, and some surgeons prefer to use separate incisions for the thoracoscope and for additional instruments such as biopsy forceps.

Collapse of the lung on the side to be explored is achieved by allowing atmospheric air to enter the pleural cavity; it is both hazardous and unnecessary to insufflate gases under pressure. A shallow pneumothorax is sometimes induced preoperatively to confirm that the lung is not adherent to the chest wall and will not be damaged when the thoracoscope is introduced.

Small effusions can be drained intraoperatively but it is prudent to drain large effusions preoperatively.

The choice of anaesthetic for thoracoscopy is rarely critical although it should be remembered that the procedure is usually short and some patients will have limited pulmonary function. An endotracheal tube is entirely adequate for control of ventilation, although better access will be possible if the lung on the operated side can be excluded from the anaesthetic circuit at will by using either one or both sides of a double-lumen tube.

OESOPHAGOSCOPY

Oesophagoscopy is used to visualize the lower pharynx and oesophagus and to provide access for extraction of foreign bodies, dilatation of strictures, injection of varices and palliative intubation of malignant tumours. A rigid oesophagoscope, inserted under general anaesthesia, gives a good view of the oesophageal mucosa and is large enough to allow the passage of biopsy forceps and dilators. The flexible, fibreoptic oesophagoscope can be used with only topical anaesthesia and light sedation, is passed more easily than the rigid instrument in patients with limited movement of the cervical spine, and can also be advanced to give a view of the stomach and proximal duodenum.

Implications of oesophageal disease

Some patients presenting for oesophagoscopy are debilitated or dehydrated as a result of dysphagia, and many are elderly so that coexistent disease is common. They are sometimes anaemic or hypoproteinaemic, the anaemia usually being caused by oesophageal bleeding. Hiatus hernia, diverticulum, stricture and achalasia predispose to reflux of gastric acid or food residues, and a low grade bronchopneumonia or even lung abscess may be present already. These factors should be assessed preoperatively and corrected if time permits (see also Chapter 9 for a more detailed discussion).

Anaesthesia for oesophagoscopy

Light premedication is all that is required, even for robust patients, because the procedure is short and coughing can be controlled easily. There is also a need for rapid return of active protective reflexes immediately after the procedure. An H_2 antagonist such as ranitidine or alternatively omeprazole can be used to raise gastric pH prior to endoscopy. These drugs do not change lower oesophageal sphincter pressure and must be given several hours before the procedure to have an effect (Chapter 9). Antacid solutions are not usually given before oesophagoscopy as they are likely to obscure the operators view. Sodium citrate is, however, a clear alternative.

Preoxygenation is followed by an intravenous induction using cricoid pressure (Sellick's manoeuvre) to control reflux of oesophageal contents. A steep head-up tilt is sometimes advocated as an additional precaution but, if there is a serious risk of aspiration (e.g. if there is active bleeding from the oesophagus), it is safer to induce anaesthesia and intubate the patient in the left lateral position. A short-acting muscle relaxant, usually suxamethonium, is given to permit intubation, preferably with a cuffed flexo-metallic tube a little on the small size for the particular patient. This should ensure least interference with the passage of the oesophagoscope, and the connecting tubing should be fastened over the front of the patient's chest for the same reason. Anaesthesia can be maintained with an inhalational agent. The patient's eyes should be protected with particular care because they are likely to be concealed by a drape around the head and the cornea will probably be damaged unless the lids are closed and secured with paper tape.

Full relaxation should be maintained until the oesophagoscope has been passed through the cricopharyngeal sphincter and, if this proves at all difficult, it may be necessary to deflate the cuff on the endotracheal tube for a few moments to provide a little more room. Spontaneous ventilation can usually be permitted, once the oesophagoscope is through the sphincter, although most anaesthetists prefer to retain control of ventilation manually with intermittent suxamethonium. Coughing during oesophagoscopy is hazardous and predisposes to oesophageal damage. Full relaxation should certainly be maintained throughout if repeated instrumentation through the cricopharyngeus is required, as in endoscopic palliative intubation of tumours. Dysrhythmias are fairly common as the oesophagoscope passes behind the heart but are rarely a source of real concern and are usually only transitory.

Recovery of consciousness should be supervised with the patient on their side, slightly head-down on a tipping trolley. Careful clinical examination and a postoperative chest X-ray are required before anything is allowed by mouth to exclude surgical emphysema, pneumoperitoneum, pneumothorax or pneumomediastinum. These signs indicate oesophageal perforation which occurs most readily if the oesophagus is acutely inflamed, or during dilatation of a tight stricture or palliative intubation through a tumour. However, it can occur during an apparently uneventful examination with either the rigid or flexible instrument, and a high degree of awareness should be maintained after any oesophagoscopy, especially if the patient complains of any discomfort on swallowing clear fluids. Exploration of the oesophagus, often involving thoracotomy, is indicated as an emergency if rupture is suspected, and may also be required if major haemorrhage results from oesophageal biopsy. Aspiration of food or acid into the lungs is a preventible complication but, if it does occur, should be treated in the usual way.

FURTHER READING

Rigid bronchoscopy

Hill A.J., Feneck R.O., Underwood S.M., Davis M.E., Marsh A. & Bromley L. (1991) The haemodynamic effects of bronchoscopy. Comparison of propofol and thiopentone with and without alfentanil pretreatment. *Anaesthesia*, **46**, 266–270.

McIntosh B.M.M., Lumley J., Morgan M. & Stradling P. (1979) Methohexitone and etomidate for bronchoscopy. *Anaesthesia*, **34**, 239–244.

Newell J.P. & Collis J.M. (1980) Anaesthesia for bronchoscopy: examination of a standard technique. *Proceedings of the Royal Society of Medicine*, **73**, 241–243.

Roberts F.L., Dixon J., Lewis G.T.R., Tackley R.M. & Prys-Roberts C. (1988) Induction and maintenance of propofol anaesthesia. A manual infusion scheme. *Anaesthesia*, **43**, 14–17.

Wark K.J., Lyons J. & Feneck R.O. (1986) The haemodynamic effects of bronchoscopy. Effect of pretreatment with fentanyl and alfentanil. *Anaesthesia*, **41**, 162–167.

Ventilation during rigid bronchoscopy

Bennetts F.E. (1977) Automatic ventilation during bronchoscopy: experience with a Bird Mark 2 ventilator. *British Journal of Anaesthesia*, **49**, 1061–1064.

Bethune D.W. & Collis J.M. (1979) Anaesthesia for bronchoscopy. *Anaesthesia*, **34**, 210–213.

Bethune D.W., Collis J.M., Burbridge N.J. & Forster D.M. (1972) Bronchoscope injectors. *Anaesthesia*, **27**, 81–83.

Borg U., Eriksson I. & Lyttkans L. *et al.* (1977) High frequency positive pressure ventilation applied in bronchoscopy under general anaesthesia. *Acta Anaesthesiologica Scandinavica* (Suppl.), **64**, 69–81.

Brendstrup A., Benkeniste D. & Pederson J.E.P. (1975) The magnitude of air admixture with a jet device in paediatric anaesthesia. *British Journal of Anaesthesia*, **47**, 390–392.

Fischer M., Seigneur F., Bourelli B., Melchior J.C., Lavoud C. & Vourch G. (1985) Jet ventilation using low or high frequencies during bronchoscopy. *British Journal of Anaesthesia*, **57**, 382–388.

Gillick J.S. (1976) Catheter inflation ventilation for bronchoscopy and laryngoscopy. *British Journal of Anaesthesia*, **46**, 612–617.

Hinds C.J., Ellis R.H. & Saloojee Y. (1978) Blood levels of nitrous oxide during bronchoscopy. *Anaesthesia*, **33**, 784–787.

Safar P. (1958) Ventilating bronchoscope. *Anesthesiology*, **19**, 406–407.

Sanders R.D. (1967) Two ventilating attachments for bronchoscopes. *Delaware Medical Journal*, **39**, 170.

Complications of rigid bronchoscopy

Gallagher M.J. & Muller B.J. (1981) Tension pneumothorax during pediatric bronchoscopy. *Anesthesiology*, **55**, 685–686.

Gupta R.K. & Barton R.P.E. (1975) Pneumothorax after general anaesthesia for panendoscopy. *British Journal of Anaesthesia*, **47**, 643.

Jenkins A.V. (1975) Electrocardiographic findings during bronchoscopy. *Anaesthesia*, **30**, 548–555.

Mette P.J. (1980) Avoiding complications during jet ventilation. *Anesthesiology*, **52**, 451–452.

Oliverio R., Ruder C.B. & Fermon C. (1979) Pneumothorax secondary to ball-valve obstruction during jet ventilation. *Anesthesiology*, **51**, 255–256.

Rosenberg P.H., Heinonen J. & Takasaki M. (1980) Lidocaine concentration in blood after topical anaesthesia of the upper respiratory tract. *Acta Anaesthesiologica Scandinavica*, **24**, 125–128.

Endobronchial laser therapy

Conacher I.D., Paes M.L. & Morritt G.N. (1985) Anaesthesia for carbondioxide laser surgery on the trachea. *British Journal of Anaesthesia*, **57**, 448–450.

George P.J.M., Garrett C.P.O., Nixon C., Hetzel M.R., Nanson E.M. & Millard F.J.C. (1987) Laser treatment for tracheobronchial tumours: local or general anaesthesia? *Thorax*, **42**, 656–660.

Hanowell L.H., Martin W.R., Savelle J.E. & Foppian L.E. (1991) Complications of general anesthesia for Nd:YAG laser resection of endobronchial tumors. *Chest*, **99**, 72–76.

Van der Spek A.L., Spargo P.M. & Norton M.L. (1988) The physics of lasers and implications for their use during airway surgery. *British Journal of Anaesthesia*, **60**, 709–729.

Fibreoptic bronchoscopy

Barr A.M. & Kurer F.L. (1984) General anaesthesia for transbronchial lung biopsy. *Anaesthesia*, **39**, 822–825.

Lett Z. & Ong G.B. (1974) Anaesthesia for flexible fibre-optic bronchoscopy. *Anaesthesia*, **29**, 623–625.

MacNaughton F.I. (1975) Anaesthesia for fibreoptic bronchoscopy. *British Journal of Anaesthesia*, **47**, 1219–1223.

Randell T., Yli-Hankala A., Valli H. & Lindgren L. (1992) Topical anaesthesia of the nasal mucosa for fibreoptic airway endoscopy. *British Journal of Anaesthesia*, **68**, 164–167.

Smith M., Calder I., Crockard A. & Nicol M.E. (1992) Oxygen saturation and cardiovascular changes during fibreoptic intubation under general anaesthesia. *Anaesthesia*, **47**, 158–161.

Smith R.B., Babinski M. & Klain M. (1977) Anaesthesia for fibreoptic bronchoscopy. *British Journal of Anaesthesia*, **49**, 193.

Bronchography

Petty C., Carden W. & Hubbarb B. (1974) Anesthetic technique to simplify and improve bronchography in children. *Radiology* **112**, 222.

Ryan D.W. (1980) Anaesthesia for bronchography in small children. *Annals of the Royal College of Surgeons*, **62**, 223–227.

Mediastinoscopy and mediastinotomy

Carlens E. (1959) Mediastinoscopy. A method for inspection and tissue biopsy in the superior mediastinum. *Diseases of the Chest*, **36**, 343–352.

Goldstraw P. (1992) The practice of cardiothoracic surgeons in the perioperative staging of non-small cell lung cancer (Editorial). *Thorax*, **47**, 1–2.

Jolly P.C., Wei-I L. & Anderson R.P. (1980) Anterior and cervical mediastinoscopy for determining operability and predicting resectability in lung cancer. *Journal of Thoracic and Cardiovascular Surgery*, **79**, 366–371.

Kliern S.G. & Savic B. (1979) Complications of mediastinoscopy. *Endoscopy*, **1**, 9–12.

Petty C. (1979) Right radial artery pressure during mediastinoscopy. *Anesthesia and Analgesia*, **58**, 428–30.

Vaughan R.S. (1978) Anaesthesia for mediastinoscopy. *Anaesthesia*, **33**, 195–198.

Vueghs P.J.M., Schurink G.A., Vaes L. & Langmemeyer J.M. (1992) Anesthesia in repeat mediastinoscopy. A retrospective study of 101 patients. *Journal of Cardiothoracic and Vascular Anesthesia*, **6**, 193–195.

Thoracoscopy

Baumgartner W.A. & Mark B.D. (1980) The use of thoracoscopy in the diagnosis of pleural disease. *Archives of Surgery*, **115**, 420–421.

Boushy S.F., North L.B. & Helgason A.H. (1978) Thoracoscopy: technique and results in eighteen patients with pleural effusion. *Chest*, **74**, 386–389.

Chui P.T., Gin T. & Chung S.C.S. (1992) Anaesthesia for a patient undergoing transthoracic endoscopic vagotomy. *British Journal of Anaesthesia*, **68**, 318–320.

Oesophagoscopy

Aitkenhead A.R. (1987) Anaesthesia for oesophageal surgery. In: Gothard J.W.W. (ed.) *Thoracic Anaesthesia. Clinical Anaesthesiology*, Vol. 1, pp. 181–205. Baillière Tindall, London.

Angorm I.B. & Hegarty M.M. (1979) Palliative pulsion intubation in oesophageal carcinoma. *Annals of the Royal College of Surgeons*, **61**, 212–214.

Kestin I.G., Chapman J.M. & Coates M.B. (1989) Alfentanil used to supplement propofol infusions for oesophagoscopy and bronchoscopy. *Anaesthesia*, **44**, 994–996.

Ward M.E., Davies T.D.W. & Strunin L. (1976) Anaesthesia for injection of bleeding oesophageal varices. *Annals of the Royal College of Surgeons*, **58**, 315–317.

4: Principles of Anaesthesia for Thoracotomy

ANATOMY OF THE TRACHEOBRONCHIAL TREE

The detailed anatomy of the tracheobronchial tree is well described in a number of standard texts and only information of specific relevance to thoracic anaesthesia will be considered here.

The adult trachea is approximately 11–12 cm in length and extends from the lower border of the cricoid cartilage at the level of the sixth cervical vertebra to its bifurcation opposite the manubrio-sternal joint and the upper border of the fifth thoracic vertebra. It is a U-shaped structure, flattened posteriorly, with an internal diameter of approximately 1.5 cm in females and 2 cm in males.

The right main bronchus is wider than the left and diverges from the trachea at an angle of only 25° as compared with 45° on the left. The two main bronchi divide into lobar branches, three on the right supplying the upper, middle and lower lobes, and two on the left for the upper and lower lobes. The early divisions are fairly constant in pattern but abnormalities do occur, usually in relation to the right upper lobe and its subdivisions. The most common of these is a supernumary bronchus originating from the right main bronchus above the right upper lobe and this, or the apical branch to the upper lobe, occasionally arises directly from the trachea.

The right middle lobe bronchus originates from the anterior aspect of the main bronchus, approximately 3 cm beyond the upper lobe orifice, and the apical segment of the right lower lobe is supplied by a posteriorly situated division which arises opposite or only a little below the right middle lobe orifice.

The upper lobe bronchus on the left side is formed by the bifurcation of the main bronchus approximately 5 cm beyond the carina and, after proceeding laterally for 1.5 cm or less, it divides into a descending branch which supplies the lingula and an ascending branch which subdivides into the segmental bronchi of the upper lobe. The left lower lobe bronchus continues from the bifurcation of the main bronchus in a downward and backward direction but, as on the right, the apical division is a separate branch arising within a centimetre of the origin.

The segmental bronchi each supply a similarly named bronchopulmonary segment and their distribution is illustrated in Fig. 4.1. These segments form the basis for surgical dissection within the lung and they receive an arterial blood supply which usually follows the same pattern. However, the lymphatic and venous drainage is more variable and usually communicates with adjacent areas of lung.

Clinical implications of tracheobronchial anatomy

In spite of the cartilage supporting its walls, the trachea is vulnerable to external injury (particularly in the neck), to compression, and to invasion by tumour which is usually an extension of a primary bronchial or laryngeal carcinoma and only rarely originates from the trachea itself. Injuries which damage or destroy tracheal cartilage may heal with the formation of a stricture; this is a well recognized complication of a prolonged intubation of tracheostomy as well as other injuries.

The detailed anatomy of the bronchial tree below the tracheal bifurcation influences the location of certain disease processes and the ease with which endobronchial instrumentation can be used to isolate the various lobes. Foreign bodies inhaled by an upright subject are more likely to enter the right main bronchus because it is wider and more in line with the trachea. In a supine subject the apical segments of the lower lobes are most at risk, whereas it is the upper lobe orifices which are gravitationally dependent in the lateral position. The right middle lobe bronchus is particularly prone to obstruction by glands because it lies in the lymphatic pathway from the right lower lobe and is surrounded by glands draining both the middle and lower lobes. Recurrent collapse, infection and ultimately bronchiectasis of the middle lobe are the results of stenosis of the middle lobe orifice caused by glandular enlargement, widely known as 'Brock's middle lobe syndrome'.

Instruments as well as accidental foreign bodies pass more readily into the

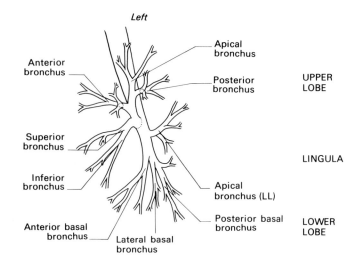

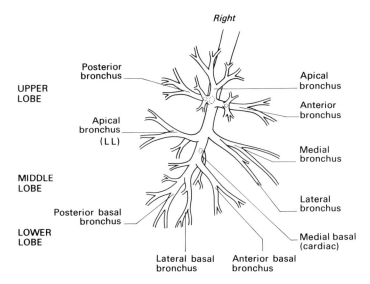

Fig. 4.1 Anatomy of the tracheobronchial tree. LL, lower lobe.

right main bronchus but endobronchial intubation on this side will obstruct the right upper lobe orifice unless there is an aperture in the bronchial cuff. The placement of an endobronchial blocker is also difficult on the right.

Although the left main bronchus is slightly more difficult to enter, endobronchial apparatus was first designed for this side because there are no subdivisions within the first 5 cm. An endobronchial blocker can be used to

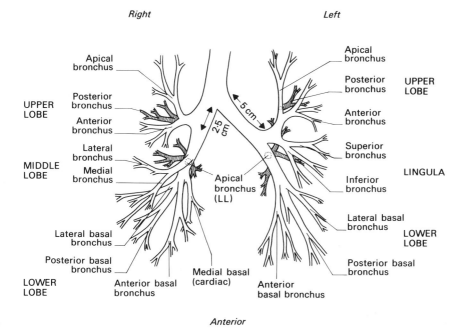

Fig. 4.1 (continued)

isolate either the upper or lower lobe on this side, but it is usually impossible to block either the left upper lobe or the lingula without affecting the other because of the common origin and close relationship of their bronchi.

Tracheobronchial anatomy in children

The dimensions of the trachea at birth and its development with age are shown in Table 4.1. The child's larynx lies more proximally than in the adult: the cricoid is at the level of the lower border of the fourth cervical vertebra in a neonate, is opposite the fifth cervical vertebra by the age of 6 years and the adult relationship is reached by the age of 13.

The bifurcation of the neonatal trachea is usually at the level of the third thoracic vertebra but can be as low as the fourth. A study on cadavers suggested that the main bronchi of children less than 3 years of age diverge from the trachea at an angle of approximately 55°. However, Bush (1963) studied children of a similar age and showed that straight suction catheters are much more likely to enter the right than the left main bronchus, as in the adult. Current opinion favours the view that the disposition of the two main bronchi is probably the same at all ages.

Table 4.1 Tracheal dimensions

Age	Length of trachea (cm)	Diameter of trachea (cm)	
		Sagittal	Coronal
Neonate	4	0.5	0.6
6–8 years	5.5	1	1.1
14–16 years	7	1	1.3
Adult	11–12	1.6–2	1.4

An important difference between child and adult is that the cricoid is the narrowest part of the larynx in childhood rather than the vocal cords as in the adult. Trauma from an endotracheal tube which passes the cords easily but fits tightly in the cricoid is followed by oedema, and a circumferential ring of epithelial oedema 1 mm thick will decrease the cross-sectional area in a neonate by 75% at the cricoid (4 mm in diameter) and by 56% in the trachea (6 mm in diameter). The small size of the child's tracheobronchial tree and the ease with which even a minor degree of trauma can cause sufficient oedema to occlude or seriously diminish the lumen precludes the use of cuffed endotracheal tubes or specialized endobronchial apparatus. However, one-lung anaesthesia can be achieved with an uncuffed tube even in infants, and Fogarty embolectomy catheters are used as blockers in paediatric practice.

SPONTANEOUS VENTILATION AND THE OPEN HEMITHORAX

Many of the anxieties associated with anaesthesia for thoracic surgery are based on historical circumstances which no longer apply. Chief amongst these were the respiratory and cardiovascular implications of spontaneous breathing during deep inhalational anaesthesia while one side of the chest was open.

When a normal subject breathes spontaneously at atmospheric pressure, the inward recoil of the lungs is exactly balanced by the outward recoil of the chest wall, and the resultant is a negative pressure of 3–5 cmH$_2$O in the potential space within the pleural cavity. This equilibrium is destroyed as soon as the chest wall and parietal pleura are opened widely on one side, and the consequences are usually quoted as pulmonary, paradoxical respiration, pendulum movement of air (*Pendelluft*), mediastinal displacement and a variety of reflex disturbances. Many of these changes reflect the dissimilar pressure on the two sides of the thorax and they are exaggerated by any factor which increases this inequality of pressure; for example, greater inspiratory effort because of respiratory insufficiency or obstruction, or active, forceful expiration against an obstruction.

Collapse of the lung will occur provided there are no adhesions, the bronchus is patent and the elastic recoil of the lung is normal. There may be little change in the size of an emphysematous lung, even when the bronchus is widely patent, because elastic recoil is diminished. The volume of lung on the intact side will decrease too, partly because the effect of gravity on the mediastinum will compress the dependent lung in the lateral position, but also because the negative pressure in the intact hemithorax will tend to draw the mediastinum to that side. Mediastinal movement is more noticeable in some animals than in man, and is more marked in the very young than in the old because the mobility of the mediastinal structures diminishes with age.

Although the conditions of the lung and the size of the opening in the chest wall govern the extent to which collapse occurs on the operated side, spontaneous breathing is likely to result in paradoxical respiration: inflation of the lung during expiration and deflation during inspiration. The term 'internal paradox' is sometimes used to distinguish this movement of the lung from 'external paradox' which is inward rather than outward movement of the rib cage during inspiration with the converse movement occurring during expiration.

Paradoxical respiration (internal paradox) can be understood most easily by considering the changes in pressure on the two sides of the chest when one pleural cavity is open to atmospheric pressure and the other is intact. An inspiratory effort exaggerates the negative pressure in the intact hemithorax but the pressure on the other side remains unchanged. As a result, gas is drawn down the trachea into the lung on the intact side, the mediastinum is displaced even further to that side, more air is drawn into the open hemithorax, and some gas may also be drawn from the collapsed lung, so causing it to deflate during inspiration. This process is reversed in expiration and it is theoretically possible for some gas to pass to and fro between the two lungs — the so-called 'pendulum air'. The extent to which this actually occurs is questionable, even when the chest is widely open on one side, but the other unequivocal sequelae of spontaneous respiration with an open hemithorax are sufficient cause for hypoxia, increased respiratory effort, and, ultimately, hypercarbia too.

Mediastinal movement is slight during quiet spontaneous respiration with an open hemithorax but is exaggerated if respiratory effort increases when it can interfere with cardiac filling and cause hypotension. Dysrhythmias are likely too because of mechanical disturbance, hypotension or respiratory insufficiency. Other reflex responses may occur during thoracotomy. Acute lung deflation in conscious subjects causes an increase in respiratory rate and increased electrical activity in some inspiratory muscles. This is thought to be a specific deflation reflex rather than the effect of hypoxia or mediastinal displacement. Manipulation of the mediastinum, and particularly dissection around the hilum of the lung, provokes vagally mediated bradycardia, hypotension, bronchoconstriction and an increase in bronchial secretion. Some protection can be afforded by the anaesthetic technique, either by blocking the vagus with atropine, by infiltrating the hilar structures with local anaesthetic, or because of the bronchodilator effect of some inhalational anaesthetics.

A moment's thought will confirm that collapse of the lung, paradoxical respiration, movement of pendulum air, and mediastinal displacement other than that attributable to gravity can all be eliminated by controlled ventilation, and the improved gas exchange which results lessens the likelihood of dysrhythmias.

CONTROLLED VENTILATION DURING THORACOTOMY

The dependent lung of a spontaneously breathing, unanaesthetized subject in the lateral thoracotomy position is better ventilated than the upper, non-dependent lung. This is because the dependent diaphragm is pushed higher into the chest at the end of expiration by the mediastinum and abdominal contents and so it contracts more effectively on inspiration. Increased ventilation is matched by improved perfusion, pulmonary blood flow increasing to the lower lung because of the effect of gravity on the low pressure pulmonary circulation.

During anaesthesia, even in the spontaneously breathing subject, the above situation changes. There is a reduction in functional residual capacity (FRC) and both lungs lose volume. As a result the position of the lungs on the pressure–volume curve changes (Fig. 4.2). The non-dependent lung now moves to a steeper part of the curve, and therefore receives more ventilation. The end result of these changes is that the upper, non-dependent lung is preferentially ventilated whilst increased pulmonary blood flow continues to the lower lung in the lateral position.

Paralysis and intermittent positive pressure ventilation (IPPV) are employed during anaesthesia for thoracic surgery in order to overcome the problem of the open pneumothorax. The compliance of the non-dependent lung remains higher than that of the lower lung during IPPV and there is

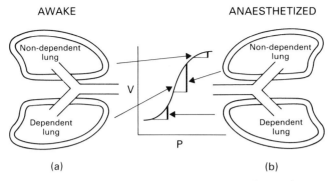

Fig. 4.2 Diagram showing the distribution of ventilation in the awake patient in the lateral decubitus position (a) and in the anaesthetized patient (b) in a similar position (Benumof J.L. *Anaesthesia for Theracic Surgery.* WB Saunders, London. 1987).

further loss of diaphragmatic tone, so that preferential ventilation to the upper lung increases. Ventilation to the non-dependent lung is likely to be increased further when the upper hemithorax is opened surgically.

One-lung ventilation is used at various times during thoracotomy in order to improve surgical access to the non-ventilated lung. This eliminates preferential ventilation to the upper lung but creates ventilation/perfusion mismatch of a much greater magnitude.

Physiology of one-lung anaesthesia

Oxygenation

Pulmonary blood flow continues to the upper lung during one-lung anaesthesia creating a 'true' shunt ($\dot{V}/\dot{Q} = 0$) in a lung where there is blood flow the alveoli but no ventilation. The blood to the upper lung ceases to take up oxygen after the first few minutes of lung collapse and therefore retains its poorly oxygenated mixed venous composition. This blood will mix with oxygenated blood in the left atrium (from the ventilated lung) causing venous admixture and lowering arterial oxygen tension.

It must not be assumed that an increase in true shunt is the only cause of an increase in venous admixture during one-lung anaesthesia. The dependent lung will be receiving the entire minute ventilation and a substantial proportion of the cardiac output. Some areas in the dependent lung are likely to be ventilated better than others, as during any general anaesthetic, and so an excess of perfusion relative to ventilation within the lung also contributes to venous admixture. The effect on arterial oxygenation of all venous admixture is exaggerated when the cardiac output is reduced because the oxygen content of mixed venous blood is lower than normal. Total venous admixture can be calculated from the shunt equation (Table 4.2) which estimates what proportion of the pulmonary blood flow would have bypassed ventilated alveoli to produce the arterial blood gas values.

Table 4.2 Shunt equation

$$\frac{\dot{Q}s}{\dot{Q}t} = \frac{\text{flow through shunt}}{\text{cardiac output}} = \frac{C\acute{c}O_2 - CaO_2}{C\acute{c}O_2 - C\overline{v}O_2}$$

where $C\acute{c}O_2$ = oxygen content in pulmonary end-capillary blood, and CaO_2, $C\overline{v}O_2$ = oxygen content of arterial and mixed venous blood.

In reported series (Table 4.3) venous admixture increases from a baseline value of approximately 20% during two-lung ventilation to a level of 30–40% during one-lung ventilation. The arterial oxygen tension (Pao_2) can be kept in the safe region of 9–16 kPa during one-lung anaesthesia in the majority of patients, with an inspired oxygen concentration between 50–100%. In individuals, however, the arterial oxygen tension may fall considerably lower than these values despite a high inspired oxygen concentration. This variation, which is not surprising considering the number of interrelated physiological factors that come into play, is discussed below.

Carbon dioxide clearance

The consequences of one-lung anaesthesia cannot be dismissed without considering the effects of carbon dioxide clearance, although these are far less in both magnitude and importance than changes in oxygenation.

There is a very slight increase in dead space when the pleura is opened during controlled ventilation in the lateral position and only minor changes when ventilation is restricted to one lung in patients undergoing pulmonary resection. The minute volume required for carbon dioxide clearance during one-lung ventilation is the same as that required when both lungs are ventilated. Only small changes in arterial carbon dioxide concentration should be expected if the pattern of ventilation is adjusted to maintain the highest possible arterial oxygen tension.

Table 4.3 Mean percentage shunt before and during one-lung ventilation in different clinical studies which are listed in alphabetical order* (Kerr, 1987). (*See also* Further Reading list)

Study	Year	Anaesthetic agent	No. of patients	Mean % shunt TLV	OLV
Aalto-Setala *et al.*	1975	Halothane	9	20	36
Bachand *et al.*	1975	Halothane	18	26	38
Capan *et al.*	1980	Halothane	21	26	38
Fiser *et al.*	1982	Halothane	85	18	30
Katz *et al.*	1982	Halothane	17	22	35
Kerr *et al.*	1974	Halothane	14	12	32
Peltola *et al.*	1983	Enflurane (2%)	12	32	49
		Enflurane (1%)	10	16	30
		Enflurane (1%)	10	19	40
Rees *et al.*	1982	Enflurane	12	18	39
Rees *et al.*	1984	Enflurane	12	20	41
		Ketamine	12	17	40
Rogers & Wansbrough	1985	Intravenous	20	21	32
Torda & Gaines	1974	Halothane	20	19	36
Weinrech & Benumof	1980	Ketamine	30	14	36

*Patients in the above studies were ventilated with almost 100% oxygen at zero end expiratory pressure and without gas being insufflated to the unventilated lung. Where there are repeated measurements the results quoted are those collected between 15 and 30 minutes after lung deflation. TLV, two-lung ventilation; OLV, one-lung ventilation

Blood flow to the non-ventilated lung

Hypoxic pulmonary vasoconstriction

In certain clinical and pathological conditions the phenomenon of hypoxic pulmonary vasoconstriction occurs in the vasculature of poorly oxygenated alveoli. The normal response of the pulmonary vasculature to atelectasis is an increase in pulmonary vascular resistance and this is thought to be due mainly to hypoxic pulmonary vasoconstriction, although a further decrease in blood flow may be due to mechanical effects of atelectasis on lung blood vessels. Hypoxic pulmonary vasoconstriction minimizes hypoxaemia by diverting blood away from poorly oxygenated alveoli to better ventilated areas of lung. The precise mechanism of hypoxic vasoconstriction remains unknown but it may be that an endothelial constrictor substance is released at alveolar level in response to hypoxia. Alternatively, hypoxia may inhibit an endothelial relaxation substance.

Many factors inhibit hypoxic pulmonary vasoconstriction. Several of these factors including vasodilator therapy, high or low pulmonary vascular pressures, hypocapnia, volatile anaesthetic agents and handling of the lung are of particular relevance to one-lung anaesthesia. Most inhalational anaesthetic agents, including halothane, enflurane and isoflurane appear to inhibit hypoxic pulmonary vasoconstriction in isolated and physiologically well controlled animal experiments. Intravenous anaesthetic agents and analgesic drugs on the other hand do not seem to inhibit hypoxic pulmonary vasoconstriction in animal preparations. In man, however, it has not been convincingly demonstrated that inhalational agents inhibit hypoxic pulmonary vasoconstriction during one-lung anaesthesia. The majority of workers have also been unable to demonstrate a reduction in shunt value when a total intravenous anaesthetic technique was used to maintain anaesthesia rather than an inhalational agent.

Hypoxic pulmonary vasoconstriction therefore seems, on current evidence, to play little role in reducing hypoxaemia during the time it takes to complete the average lobectomy or pneumonectomy. Volatile anaesthetic agents do not significantly impair arterial oxygenation during one-lung anaesthesia and remain the primary anaesthetic agent of choice for thoracotomy.

Preoperative lung function

Diseased lung may have considerably reduced blood supply as a result of hypoxic pulmonary vasoconstriction or, in some instances, for physical reasons such as collapse/consolidation or infiltration by tumour. Certain patients with poor lung function are accepted for lung resection on the basis that their diseased lung is contributing little to gas exchange. If this type of pulmonary disease is largely confined to the side of surgery then one-lung ventilation may have little effect on pulmonary gas exchange. Nomoto (1987) used a lung perfusion scanning technique to calculate the perfusion partition between the dependent and non-dependent lung prior to surgery and found that this correlated with arterial oxygenation during one-lung ventilation. The ratio was as high as 85% in patients with empyema, some of whom had extremely low blood flow to the diseased lung. In patients with carcinoma the perfusion partition ratio was 57% and this group had significantly poorer oxygenation during one-lung ventilation.

Kerr *et al.* (1974) reported that patients undergoing non-resection procedures, such as oesophageal surgery, tended to have poorer arterial oxygenation during one-lung ventilation than those undergoing lung resection. It was presumed that in the former oesophageal group a relatively normal lung was being collapsed to provide surgical access. Katz *et al.* (1982) also found that patients with a preoperative forced expired volume in 1 second (FEV_1) nearest predicted values were more likely to be hypoxic during one-lung ventilation, although others have not confirmed this.

Cardiac output

Changes in cardiac output are likely to affect arterial oxygenation during thoracic surgery. If oxygen consumption remains steady a decrease in cardiac output will cause a drop in mixed venous oxygen content. Some of this relatively desaturated blood will be shunted during one-lung anaesthesia and further exacerbate hypoxaemia. Cardiac output can fall for a number of reasons during thoracotomy. These include major blood loss, dysrhythmias, the use of high inflation pressures, the application of positive end expiratory pressure (PEEP) to the dependent lung and the use of high levels of PEEP to the lower lung combined with continuous insufflation of oxygen at a positive pressure to the upper lung. Surgical manipulation and retraction in and around the mediastinum, causing a reduction in venous return, is, however, probably the commonest cause of sudden changes in cardiac output during thoracotomy.

Management of one-lung anaesthesia

Arterial hypoxaemia is common in innumerable clinical situations and the extent to which any particular degree can be regarded as devoid of risk depends upon many factors. These include the functional state of organs such as the brain, heart and kidneys, the oxygen tension to which the individual is accustomed, the metabolic demand and whether tissue oxygenation is preserved in spite of hypoxaemia. Many variables influence the delivery of oxygen to the tissues and a minimum 'safe' value for arterial oxygen tension which is applicable to all patients, under all circumstances, cannot be quoted. In general a Pao_2 of 9 kPa or above, which corresponds to an oxygen saturation of 93.5% with a normal haemoglobin dissociation curve, is tolerable with an inspired oxygen concentration of between 50 and 100%. This, however, may be insufficient for occasional patients with vascular disease in a critical site where tissue oxygen tension is low because blood flow is reduced as well as arterial oxygen tension. Conversely, there are some patients acclimatized to chronic hypoxaemia in whom an arterial tension of 9 kPa is very difficult to achieve during thoracotomy but who, nevertheless, withstand the procedure without harm. In general terms the lower the oxygen tension is below normal values the greater the risk. The occasional incidence of acute renal failure, confusion or focal signs of neurological damage after an apparently uncomplicated thoracotomy, during which there has been no hypotension, must sometimes be attributed to hypoxaemia.

Venous admixture during one-lung ventilation in reported series (Table 4.3) varies between 30–40%, but even at this level the majority of patients will have a Pao_2 in a safe range between 9–16 kPa with an inspired oxygen concentration ranging from 50–100%. In individual patients, however, the Pao_2 will be well below this value. Hypoxia is particularly likely to occur in the following circumstances:

1 During thoracotomy for disease other than in the lung.
2 When there is significant pre-existing disease in the dependent lung.
3 Ventilation to some or all of the dependent lung is compromised by a poorly placed or partially obstructed endobronchial tube.
4 Cardiac output is low.
5 The function of the dependent lung has deteriorated during the operation for a variety of reasons including prolonged surgery and anaesthesia, a poor pattern of ventilation and massive blood transfusion.

Some of the above factors are amenable to control and will be discussed in the following section. Often the exact cause of hypoxia is not immediately obvious but the essential principle of ventilation during one-lung anaesthesia is to match ventilation to pulmonary blood flow as far as possible and thereby minimize the shunt. This is discussed below.

Elimination of the pulmonary shunt

Surgical occlusion of the pulmonary vessels early in a lung resection procedure will obviously minimize any period of potential hypoxia. It is rarely possible to achieve this, however, and once the surgeon is in a position to control and divide vessels the period of one-lung anaesthesia is almost over. It is not established practice, nor regarded as necessary, to dissect out and clamp pulmonary vessels during non-resection operations such as oesophagectomy.

Inspired gas mixture

An inspired oxygen concentration of at least 50% should be used during one-lung ventilation. This may well provide satisfactory arterial oxygen concentrations in the majority of patients and can sensibly be administered in an air/oxygen mixture with the addition of an inhalational agent such as isoflurane. It may be necessary to increase the inspired oxygen concentration from the baseline 50% up to 100% if arterial oxygen saturations remain low and other ventilatory manoeuvres (see below) are ineffective in improving the situation. This will improve oxygenation because of the increased uptake of oxygen from the alveoli with low ventilation/perfusion ratios in the dependent lung. Many anaesthetists prefer to use 100% inspired oxygen concentration from the outset, however, believing that the advantages of a greater margin of safety far outweigh potential problems of absorption collapse. It is difficult to challenge this approach.

Pattern of ventilation

As previously discussed, carbon dioxide elimination is rarely a problem provided the same minute volume is maintained during one-lung anaesthesia as was employed during two-lung ventilation. Ventilator settings are then adjusted to provide adequate alveolar ventilation in the dependent lung without an excessive rise in mean intra-alveolar pressure which will only serve to divert the low pressure pulmonary blood flow away to the non-ventilated upper lung. An initial tidal volume of approximately 10 ml/kg is set to provide adequate ventilation with a peak inspiratory pressure of $30 \, cmH_2O$ or less. It may be necessary to increase or decrease this tidal volume, and occasionally high inflation pressures have to be tolerated for a short period of time. Much will depend on the compliance of the lower lung. If inflation pressures remain in excess of $35 \, cmH_2O$ despite adjusting the tidal volume down to 600 ml or so in the average 70–80 kg adult it is worth reassessing the position of the double-lumen tube. Is a right-sided tube obstructing the upper lobe orifice, for example? Is a long left-sided tube impinging on the left upper lobe orifice? It may be necessary to reposition the tube or aspirate secretions from the dependent lung in order to lower peak inflation pressures.

Long inspiratory times reduce peak inflation pressure and improve the distribution of gas in the ventilated lung but increase the mean intra-alveolar pressure. In this situation blood flow may also be diverted away from the lower lung so it is preferable to use a conventional, fairly short, inspiratory time with a ratio of inspiration to expiration of 1 : 2. Once a satisfactory initial pattern of ventilation has been established one-lung anaesthesia can be monitored by continuous pulse oximetry and intermittent blood gas analysis (see Chapter 5).

Manual ventilation

Most authors do not report any improvement in arterial oxygen tension if manual ventilation rather than mechanical ventilation is used during one-lung anaesthesia, and it is all too easy to achieve an unnecessarily high minute volume when ventilating by hand. It is useful however to ventilate by hand while the pleura is being opened or closed to prevent damage to underlying lung. Manual ventilation may also be requested to test the integrity of bronchial suture lines at a known pressure, to increase ventilation to the operated lung so that tissue planes and fissures can be delineated more clearly, and to re-inflate areas of collapse, particularly to ensure full expansion of the residual lobe or lung before the chest is closed. Manual ventilation may also be preferred throughout for thoracic surgery in infants.

A few breaths of manual ventilation, delivering a large tidal volume to the dependent lung, followed by endobronchial suction may result in a significant improvement in arterial oxygen tension if this has fallen because of atelectasis. The simple manoeuvre of temporarily re-inflating the upper lung with 100% oxygen has also been shown to improve oxygenation. Over-vigorous manual ventilation, however, can lower arterial oxygen tension because of adverse effects on both cardiac output and the distribution of pulmonary blood flow caused by an increase in intra-alveolar pressure in the dependent lung.

Positive end expiratory pressure

Positive end expiratory pressure (PEEP) may prevent atelectasis in the dependent lung but this is achieved at the expense of diverting blood flow away from that lung and also reducing cardiac output. Most studies (Fig. 4.3) have failed to demonstrate any benefit when PEEP is applied to the dependent lung during one-lung anaesthesia. PEEP can, however, be beneficial in individual patients and may be worth introducing in certain circumstances with careful monitoring by pulse oximetry and blood gas analysis.

Insufflation of oxygen at positive pressure

Delivery of oxygen to the upper lung by insufflation at a positive pressure of $5–10\,cmH_2O$ (similar to continuous positive airway pressure, CPAP) will improve arterial oxygenation because additional oxygen is taken up by the pulmonary blood flow to the previously non-ventilated lung (Fig. 4.4). This

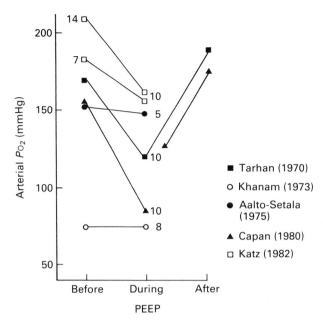

Fig. 4.3 Effect of positive end expiratory pressure (PEEP) applied to the dependent lung during one-lung ventilation (OLV) on arterial oxygenation. The results are taken from clinical studies indicated by first authors (see Further Reading section). Figures in the centre section refer to the positive pressure applied and those in the left section indicate the tidal volume (ml/kg) (Kerr, 1987).

technique is not widely used in the UK, although it is relatively simple to apply. It may be particularly useful during oesophageal surgery when the left lung is deflated because, as previously discussed, this group of patients is more likely to be hypoxic during one-lung anaesthesia.

PEEP combined with CPAP

PEEP applied to the dependent lung combined with oxygen delivered to the upper lung at a positive pressure certainly improves measurements of arterial oxygenation because the deleterious effect of pulmonary blood flow diversion is negated with this technique. Cardiac output, however, can be substantially reduced by this technique so that total oxygen delivery may not be improved (Cohen *et al.*, 1988). Most anaesthetists working with a relatively fast surgeon find the disadvantages of this technique outweigh any potential short-term advantages.

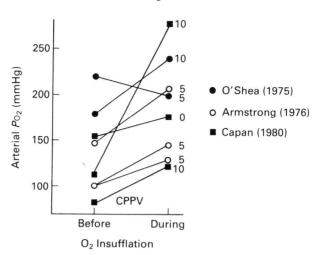

Fig. 4.4 Effect on arterial oxygen tension of insufflating oxygen into the unventilated lung during one-lung ventilation. Results are taken from clinical studies indicated by first authors (see Further Reading section). Figures next to the symbols refer to any positive pressure applied. CPPV, continuous positive pressure ventilation (Kerr, 1987).

High frequency jet ventilation

High frequency jet ventilation (HFJV) can be used to provide satisfactory gas exchange during thoracotomy either via an endotracheal tube or some form of endobronchial tube. The elegant study of El Baz *et al.* (1982) (Fig. 4.5) showed how effective HFJV can be during thoracic surgery when applied via a single-lumen endobronchial tube and a number of anaesthetists use some form of HFJV on a routine basis during thoracotomy. Despite the fact that some authors advocate the use of HFJV during thoracotomy and one-lung anaesthesia it has not been widely adopted clinically. Jenkins *et al.* (1987) reported that, although surgical conditions and gas exchange were satisfactory with the use of HFJV during thoracotomy, it was difficult to assess adequacy of ventilation. Howland *et al.* (1987) found that surgical access was hindered by overdistension of the upper lung during HFJV. Neither of the above groups recommended HFJV for routine clinical practice.

HFJV may well have a role to play in more specialized circumstances and it has been advocated for a variety of procedures including bilateral bullectomy, the management of bronchopleural fistula, sleeve resection of the right upper lobe and airway surgery. These applications are discussed in the appropriate chapters which follow Chapter 6.

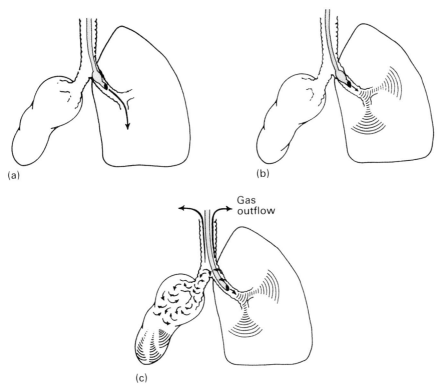

(a)   (b)

Gas outflow

(c)

Fig. 4.5 High frequency jet ventilation with an uncuffed endobronchial tube. (a) OL-IPPV: conventional one-lung ventilation ($\dot{Q}s/\dot{Q}t$ 37%; PaO_2 141 mmHg). (b) OL-HFV: high frequency jet ventilation to the dependent lung ($\dot{Q}s/\dot{Q}t$ 31%; PaO_2 235 mmHg). (c) MOL-HFV: high frequency jet ventilation to the dependent lung with the bronchial cuff deflated, allowing insufflation of gas to the upper lung ($\dot{Q}s/\dot{Q}t$ 19%; PaO_2 379 mmHg). (El Baz *et al.* 1982.)

FURTHER READING

Anatomy of the tracheobronchial tree

Brock R.C. (1954) *The Anatomy of the Bronchial Tree with Special Reference to the Surgery of Lung Abscess*, 2nd edn. Oxford University Press, Oxford.

Burri P.H. & Weibel E.R. (1977) Ultrastructure and morphometry of the developing lung. In: Hodson W.A. (ed.) *The Development of the Lung*. Marcel Dekker, New York.

Bush G.H. (1963) Tracheo-bronchial suction in infants and children. *British Journal of Anaesthesia*, **35**, 322–326.

Eckenhoff J.E. (1951) Some anatomic considerations of the infant larynx influencing endotracheal anaesthesia. *Anesthesiology*, **12**, 401–405.

Kubota Y., Toyoda Y., Nagata N. *et al.* (1986) Tracheobronchial angles in infants and children. *Anesthesiology*, **64**, 374–376.

Landing B.H. (1979) Congenital malformations and genetic disorders of the respiratory tract. *American Review of Respiratory Disease*, **120**, 151–185.

Miller W.S. (1950) *The Lung*, 2nd edn. Charles C. Thomas, Springfield, Illinois. Thoracic Society (1950) The nomenclature of broncho-pulmonary anatomy. *Thorax*, **5**, 222–228.

Spontaneous ventilation and the open hemithorax

Aviado D.M. (1975) Regulation of bronchomotor tone during anesthesia. *Anesthesiology*, **42**, 68–80.

Brauer L. (1906) *Uber Pneumothorax*. Marburg.

Guz A., Noble M.I.M., Eislele J.H. & Trenchard D. (1971) The effect of lung deflation on breathing man. *Clinical Science*, **40**, 451–461.

Maloney J.V., Schmutzer K.J. & Raschke E. (1961) Paradoxical respiration and 'pendelluft'. *Journal of Thoracic and Cardiovascular Surgery*, **41**, 291–298.

Nosworthy M.D. (1941) Controlled respiration and cyclopropane. *Proceedings of the Royal Society of Medicine*, **34**, 479–483.

Physiology of one-lung anaesthesia

Aalto-Setala M., Heinonen J. & Salorinne Y. (1975) Cardiorespiratory function during thoracic anaesthesia: a comparison of two-lung ventilation and one-lung ventilation with and without $PEEP_5$. *Acta Anaesthesiologica Scandinavica*, **19**, 287–295.

Armstrong R.F., Hutchinson J.M., Lincoln C.R., Ingram D. & Soutter L. (1976) Continuous measurement of arterial oxygen tension during one-lung anaesthesia. *British Journal of Anaesthesia*, **48**, 1005–1010.

Augustine S.D. & Benumof J.L. (1984) Halothane and isoflurane do not impair oxygenation during one-lung anaesthesia in patients undergoing thoracotomy. *Anesthesiology*, **61**, A484.

Aviado D.M. (1960) Effects of acute atelectasis on lobar blood flow. *American Journal of Physiology*, **198**, 349–353.

Bachand R., Audet J., Meloche R. & Denis R. (1975) Physiological changes associated with unilateral pulmonary ventilation during operations on the lung. *Canadian Anaesthetists' Society Journal*, **22**, 659–664.

Benumof J.L. (1985) One lung ventilation and hypoxic pulmonary vasoconstriction: implications for anaesthetic management. *Anesthesia and Analgesia*, **64**, 821–833.

Benumof J.L. (1986) Isoflurane anesthesia and arterial oxygenation during one-lung ventilation (Editorial). *Anesthesiology*, **64**, 419–422.

Benumof J.L. & Wahrenbrock E.A. (1975) Local effects of anaesthetics on regional hypoxic pulmonary vasoconstriction. *Anesthesiology*, **43**, 525–531.

Benumof J.L., Augustine S.D. & Gibbons J.A. (1987) Halothane and isoflurane only slightly impair arterial oxygenation during one-lung ventilation in patients undergoing thoracotomy. *Anesthesiology*, **67**, 910–915.

Bjertanaes L., Hauge A. & Kriz M. (1980) Hypoxia-induced pulmonary vasoconstriction: effects of fentanyl following different routes of administration. *Acta Anaesthesiologic Scandinavica*, **24**, 53–57.

Bjertanaes L.J. & Mundal R. (1980) The pulmonary vasoconstrictor response to hypoxia during enflurane anesthesia. *Acta Anaesthesiologica Scandinavica*, **24**, 252–256.

Brown D.R., Kafer E.R., Robertson V.O., Wilcox B.R. & Murray S.F. (1977) Improved oxygenation during thoracotomy with selective PEEP to the dependent lung. *Anesthesia and Analgesia*, **56**, 26–31.

Capan L.M., Turndoff H., Patel C., Ramathan R., Acinpura A. & Chalon J. (1980) Optimization of arterial oxygenation during one-lung anesthesia. *Anesthesia and Analgesia*, **59**, 847–851.

Cohen E., Eisenkraft J.B., Thys D.M., Kirschner P.A. & Kaplan J.A. (1988) Oxygenation and haemodynamic changes during one-lung ventilation: effects of $CPAP_{10}$, $PEEP_{10}$, and $CPAP_{10}/PEEP_{10}$. *Journal of Cardiothoracic Anesthesia*, **2**, 34–40.

D'Oliveira M., Sykes M.K., Chakrabarti M.K., Orchard C. & Keslin J. (1981) Depression of hypoxic pulmonary vasoconstriction by sodium nitroprusside and nitroglycerin. *British Journal of Anaesthesia*, **53**, 11–18.

Domino K.B., Borowec L., Alexander C.M. *et al.* (1986) Influence of isoflurane on hypoxic pulmonary vasoconstriction in dogs. *Anesthesiology*, **64**, 423–429.

Fiser W.P., Friday C.D. & Read R.C. (1982) Changes in arterial oxygenation and pulmonary shunt during thoracotomy with endobronchial anesthesia. *Journal of Thoracic and Cardiovascular Surgery*, **83**, 523–531.

Hurford W.E., Kolker A.C. & Strauss H.W. (1987) The use of ventilation/perfusion scans to predict oxygenation during anesthesia. *Anesthesiology*, **67**, 841–843.

Katz J.A., Laverne R.G., Fairley H.B. & Thomas A.N. (1982) Pulmonary oxygen exchange during endobronchial anesthesia. *Anesthesiology*, **56**, 164–171.

Kerr J.H. (1987) Ventilation and blood flow during thoracic surgery. In: Gothard J.W.W. (ed.) *Thoracic Anaesthesia. Clinical Anaesthesiology*, Vol. 1, pp. 61–78. Baillière Tindall, London.

Kerr J.H., Crampton Smith A., Prys-Roberts C., Meloche R. (1973) Observations during endobronchial anaesthesia I: ventilation and carbon dioxide clearance. *British Journal of Anaesthesia*, **45**, 159–166.

Kerr J.H., Crampton Smith A., Prys-Roberts C., Meloche R. & Foëx (1974) Observations during endobronchial anaesthesia II: oxygenation. *British Journal of Anaesthesia*, **46**, 86–92.

Khanam T. & Branthwaite M.A. (1973a) Arterial oxygenation during one-lung anaesthesia (1). *Anaesthesia*, **28**, 132–138.

Khanam T. & Branthwaite M.A. (1973b) Arterial oxygenation during one-lung anaesthesia (2). *Anaesthesia*, **28**, 280–290.

Larsson A., Malmkvist G. & Werner O. (1987) Variations in lung volume and compliance during pulmonary surgery. *British Journal of Anaesthesia*, **59**, 585–591.

Malmkvist G. (1989) Maintenance of oxygenation during one-lung ventilation. Effect of intermittent reinflation of the collapsed lung with oxygen. *Anesthesia and Analgesia*, **68**, 763–766.

Nilsson E., Slater E.M. & Reenberg J. (1956) The cost of the quiet lung: fluctuations in in Pao_2 when the Carlens tube is used in pulmonary surgery. *Acta Anaesthesiologica Scandinavica*, **9**, 49–55.

Nomoto Y. (1987) Preoperative pulmonary blood flow and one-lung anaesthesia. *Canadian Journal of Anaesthesia*, **34**, 447–449.

Nunn J.F. (1961) The distribution of inspired gas during thoracic surgery. *Annals of the Royal College of Surgeons*, **28**, 223–237.

O'Shea P.J., Savage T.N. & Walton B. (1975) Effect of oxygen insufflation during one-lung anaesthesia. *Proceedings of the Royal Society of Medicine*, **68**, 772–773.

Peltola K. (1983) Central haemodynamics and oxygenation during thoracic anaesthesia. *Acta Anaesthesiologica Scandinavica* (Suppl. 77) **27**, 1–50.

Rees D.I. & Wansbrough S.R. (1982) One-lung anesthesia: percent shunt and arterial oxygen tension during continuous insufflation of oxygen to the non-ventilated lung. *Anesthesia and Analgesia*, **61**, 507–512.

Rees D.I. & Gaines G.Y. (1984) One-lung anesthesia — a comparison of pulmonary gas exchange during anesthesia with ketamine or enflurane. *Anesthesia and Analgesia*, **63**, 521–525.

Rogers S.N. & Benumof J.L. (1985) Halothane and isoflurane do not decrease Pao_2 during one-lung ventilation in intravenously anesthetized patients. *Anesthesia and Analgesia*, **64**, 946–954.

Seed R.F. (1967) The cost of the quiet lung? *Proceedings of the Royal Society of Medicine*, **60**, 750–752.

Slinger P., Triolet W. & Wilson J. (1988) Improving arterial oxygenation during one-lung ventilation. *Anesthesiology*, **68**, 291–295.

Sykes M.K., Hurtig J.B., Tait A.R. & Chakrabarti M.K. (1977a) Reduction of hypoxic pulmonary vasoconstriction during diethyl ether anaesthesia in the dog. *British Journal of Anaesthesia*, **49**, 293–298.

Sykes M.K., Hurtig J.B., Tait A.R. & Chakrabarti M.K. (1977b) Reduction of hypoxic pulmonary vasoconstriction in the dog during administration of nitrous oxide. *British Journal of Anaesthesia*, **49**, 301–307.

Tarhan S. & Lundborg R.O. (1968) Blood gas and pH studies during the use of the Carlens catheter. *Canadian Anaesthetists' Society Journal*, **15**, 458–467.

Tarhan S. & Lundborg R.O. (1970) Effects of increased expiratory pressure on blood gas tensions and pulmonary shunting during thoracotomy with the use of the Carlens catheter. *Canadian Anaesthetists' Society Journal*, **17**, 4–11.

Tarhan S. & Lundborg R.O. (1971) Carlens endobronchial catheter versus regular endotracheal tube during thoracic surgery: a comparison of blood gas tensions and pulmonary shunting. *Canadian Anaesthetists' Society Journal*, **18**, 594–599.

Thomson D.F. & Campbell D. (1973) Changes in arterial oxygen tension during one-lung anaesthesia. *British Journal of Anaesthesia*, **45**, 611–616.

Thys D.M., Cohen E. & Eisenkraft J.B. (1988) Mixed venous oxygen saturation during thoracic anesthesia. *Anesthesiology*, **69**, 1005–1009.

Torda T.A., McCulloch C.H., O'Brien H.D., Wright J.S. & Horton D.A. (1974) Pulmonary venous admixture during one-lung anaesthesia. *Anaesthesia*, **29**, 272–279.

Weinrech A.I., Silvay G. & Lumb P.D. (1980) Continuous ketamine infusion for one-lung anaesthesia. *Canadian Anaesthetists' Society Journal*, **27**, 485–490.

Werner O., Malmkvist G., Beckman A., Stahle S. & Nordstrom L. (1984a) Carbon dioxide elimination from each lung during endobronchial anaesthesia. Effects of posture and pulmonary artery pressure. *British Journal of Anaesthesia*, **56**, 995–1001.

Werner O., Malmkvist G., Beckman A., Stahle S. & Nordstrom L. (1984b) Gas exchange and haemodynamics during thoracotomy. *British Journal of Anaesthesia*, **56**, 1343–1349.

High frequency jet ventilation and thoracic surgery

El-Baz N.M., Kittle C.F., Faber L.P. & Welsher W. (1982) High-frequency ventilation with an uncuffed endobronchial tube. *Journal of Thoracic and Cardiovascular Surgery*, **84**, 823–828.

Howland W.S., Carlon G.C., Goldiner P.L. *et al.* (1987) High-frequency jet ventilation during thoracic surgical procedures. *Anesthesiology*, **67**, 1009–1012.

Jenkins J., Cameron E.W.J., Milne A.C. & Hunter R.M. (1987) One lung anaesthesia. Cardiovascular and respiratory function compared with conventional and high frequency jet ventilation. *Anaesthesia*, **42**, 938–943.

Morgan B.A., Perks D., Conacher I.D. & Paes M.L. (1987) Combined unilateral high frequency jet ventilation and contralateral intermittent positive pressure ventilation. *Anaesthesia*, **42**, 975–979.

5: Practical Management
of Anaesthesia for Thoracotomy

ANAESTHETIC TECHNIQUE

Light general anaesthesia with muscular relaxation and controlled ventilation is an ideal combination for the majority of procedures involving thoracotomy. Special considerations apply to patients with myasthenia gravis or the myasthenic syndrome (Chapter 10), a bronchopleural fistula (Chapter 7), lung cyst (Chapter 7), or a compromised airway (Chapters 9 and 10). These are discussed individually in the appropriate chapters.

Induction

Anaesthesia is induced intravenously as for most major surgery. The choice of agent is rarely important, particularly for a relatively long procedure such as lung resection, unless there is a history of asthma or drug allergy. An inhalational induction may be preferable in small children and is also indicated in certain types of upper airway obstruction (Chapter 9).

In most situations endobronchial intubation can be carried out following the administration of an adequate dose of a non-depolarizing muscle relaxant such as pancuronium for a long procedure or either atracurium or vecuronium for shorter procedures such as open lung biopsy. Suxamethonium is the preferred muscle relaxant if there is a suspicion that endobronchial intubation may be difficult, provided there are no indications that manual inflation with a mask and airway may be difficult. Suxamethonium provides rapid and profound relaxation in the patient with a full dentition and a receding mandible in whom the placement of a double-lumen tube may prove difficult. Musculoskeletal pains following the use of suxamethonium are not a significant problem after thoracotomy.

One rare feature of malignant lung disease relevant to the use of muscle relaxants is that of myopathy. Peripheral myopathy is usually associated with small cell carcinoma of the lung and is termed the myasthenic or Eaton–Lambert syndrome, after the workers who described its electromyographic features. The use of muscle relaxants in the myasthenic syndrome and in patients with myasthenia gravis is discussed in Chapter 10.

Maintenance

Intermittent positive pressure ventilation is continued following induction with an inspired gas mixture of oxygen (usually a minimum concentration of 50%) in nitrous oxide or, alternatively, an air/oxygen mixture. A volatile agent such as isoflurane or ethrane is used to augment anaesthesia (see Table 5.1). The choice of agent can be based on conventional criteria because, as discussed in Chapter 4, the effect of inhalational agents on the conduct of one-lung ventilation is minimal. It may be necessary to increase the inspired oxygen concentration to as high as 100% during one-lung ventilation and as previously discussed many anaesthetists prefer to use high inspired oxygen concentrations from the outset. In either situation the inspired concentration of volatile agent must be increased to eliminate the possibility of patient awareness.

Intravenous opioid analgesics administered at the beginning of surgery help establish adequate analgesia intraoperatively and in the immediate postoperative period. The choice of opioid used is rarely important but, as dose requirements vary widely, many patients will require additional incre-

Table 5.1 Rationale for use of volatile anaesthetic agents during thoracotomy and one-lung anaesthesia. After Benumof (1985)

1 Have bronchodilatory effect
2 Obtund airway reflexes
3 Allow the use of a high inspired oxygen concentration
4 Do not impair arterial oxygenation any more than intravenous agents
5 Are rapidly eliminated postoperatively

ments of opioid at the end of surgery prior to (or as part of) the establishment of a postoperative analgesic regime (see Chapter 6). If epidural opioids are to be used for postoperative pain relief many anaesthetists prefer not to use intravenous opioids during surgery. This would certainly be the case if the epidural was established preoperatively, or immediately after induction, rather than at the end of surgery.

MONITORING

Minimum requirements

Electrocardiography, pulse oximetry, non-invasive blood pressure measurement and inspired/expired gas analysis are basic monitoring requirements for short low-risk thoracic procedures such as mediastinoscopy. Peripheral venous access is usually adequate for minor procedures.

Major thoracic surgery

Patients undergoing more complex types of surgery, such as lung resection, will require additional monitoring. Invasive arterial pressure monitoring via a radial artery cannula provides a continuous read-out of systemic blood pressure which is extremely valuable in following sudden changes in pressure associated with surgical manipulation. An arterial line also provides a site for intermittent blood gas analysis and haemoglobin, blood sugar and electrolyte estimations both during and after surgery. Despite the relative accuracy of pulse oximetry during one-lung ventilation intermittent blood gas analysis provides a useful check of arterial oxygenation and, of course, additional information concerning respiratory and metabolic acidosis.

It is usual to insert a central venous line prior to major thoracic surgery to provide a route for rapid transfusion and the continuous measurement of central venous pressure. Our practice is to insert one or two cannulae in the internal jugular vein. These are placed in the vein on the side of surgery so that any potential complications of insertion such as pneumothorax or haemothorax will be revealed at surgery and the dependent lung will not be adversely affected. In major cases both a wide-bore (14 gauge) cannula and a triple-lumen catheter are inserted using the Seldinger technique. A multi-lumen catheter provides a reliable route for the continuous measurement of right-sided cardiac filling pressures and the infusion of drugs such as insulin, intravenous nitrates or opioids.

Pulmonary artery catheters can only be placed in the lung contralateral to surgery if radiological screening facilities are available and the pressure measurements obtained are difficult to interpret with the patient in a lateral position. For these reasons pulmonary artery catheters are infrequently used during thoracic surgery (and particularly during lung resection) in the UK. If it is considered that the measurement of pulmonary artery pressure and/or cardiac output will be useful in the postoperative period a valved sheath can be inserted into a central vein immediately after induction of anaesthesia to facilitate pulmonary artery catheterization following completion of surgery.

Heat loss may be substantial during thoracic surgery, particularly during thoraco-abdominal procedures where a vast surface area of lung, chest wall and abdominal contents are exposed to the ambient temperature of the operating theatre. Measures to minimize heat loss include raising the ambient temperature, the humidification of inspired gases, the use of a heating blanket, plastic patient drapes and the warming of transfusion fluids. Nasopharyngeal temperature, or some other central temperature, should be measured during complex and prolonged procedures. It may also be useful to measure peripheral skin temperature if skin flaps are to be raised to cover chest wall defects.

Urinary retention is common following thoracotomy but routine bladder catheterization is not usually undertaken. Bladder catheterization is indicated, however, in patients with poor renal function, those undergoing procedures with major blood and fluid loss, those in whom epidural analgesia is employed (see Chapter 6) and in patients who are electively ventilated postoperatively.

POSTURE

Thoracotomy for pulmonary or oesophageal disease is usually carried out through a lateral incision. The use of posture to control pulmonary secretions during thoracotomy is now largely of historical interest (Chapter 1), but the upright posture is still invaluable for this purpose during drainage of an acute empyema, or the induction of anaesthesia in a patient with a large bronchopleural fistula.

The lateral thoracotomy position

The patient remains supine until intubation, venous and arterial cannulation and the setting up of monitoring apparatus have been completed and is only turned into the lateral position after the side of surgery has been confirmed by the surgeon and by reference to a recent chest X-ray or the case notes.

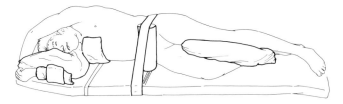

Fig. 5.1 The lateral thoracotomy position. Note the pillow between the legs and the chest and pelvic supports.

The lower shoulder is pulled through anteriorly, so allowing the flexed arm to be tucked under the pillow supporting the head. The upper arm is extended, and placed over and in front of the head to pull the scapula away from the site of operation without stretching the brachial plexus. Some surgeons, however, prefer the upper arm to be placed in an arm support attached to the head of the operating table. Stability of the pelvis is achieved by flexing the lower leg at the hip and knee while the upper leg, padded with a pillow, is kept relatively straight. Further stability can be achieved in a variety of ways. Padded rests can be placed in front of the lower sternum and pelvis and a wide strap provides additional support if placed across the pelvis, pelvic support and operating table (Fig. 5.1). Alternatively, the patient can be stabilized on a mattress which conforms to body contours and becomes rigid once its air has been evacuated (Fig. 5.2). Surgical access to the chest can be improved if the patient's lower thorax is placed directly over a section of the operating table which can be raised to aid distraction of the ribs of the upper chest (see also Fig. 5.2). This section of the operating table is lowered prior to chest closure.

After the patient has been turned, it is essential to confirm, either by auscultation or with the fibreoptic bronchoscope, that the endobronchial tube has not been displaced. Endobronchial tubes can be displaced onwards

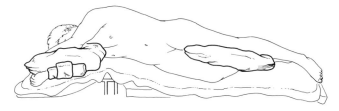

Fig. 5.2 The lateral thoracotomy position with a patient stabilized by a conformable mattress. Note the 'bridge' raised in the operating table, directly below the chest, to aid surgical access.

into the bronchial tree if the neck is flexed (see section on the selection and use of double-lumen endobronchial tubes, p. 98), and can then obstruct a lobar bronchus, even on the left side. Double-lumen tubes may also kink in the pharynx unless the head is kept slightly extended on the neck. Finally, it should be ascertained that the patient's eyes are taped and all potential pressure points are padded.

CHEST CLOSURE
AND TERMINATION OF ANAESTHESIA

The aim at the end of any operation in the thoracic cavity must be to achieve full expansion of all remaining lung tissue, and the mediastinum should remain as central as possible. It is usually necessary to insert chest drainage tubes towards the end of surgery to drain the pleural cavity so that air or fluid cannot accumulate. The lung is re-expanded as fully as possible once the drains are in place and also before the chest is closed. Manual re-inflation is helpful at this stage and re-expansion of atelectatic areas will be achieved more easily if the surgeon restrains well expanded areas so that the ventilating gas is driven to the atelectatic areas. A short period of ventilation to the surgical or upper lung alone also aids this process. The chest drainage tubes are connected to an underwater seal bottle or collecting device and suction is usually applied to this container (but *not* in the case of pneumonectomy). The application and management of chest drainage are described in more detail in Chapter 6.

After completion of surgery, and closure of the chest wall, anaesthesia is lightened and spontaneous respiration re-established in the usual manner, unless postoperative ventilation is planned. Prior to removal of the endobronchial tube the patient is placed in a supine position and any secretions or debris suctioned from both lungs. The tube is then removed following manual re-expansion of the lungs. Certain types of oesophageal surgery, such as oesophagectomy with colonic interposition, can lead to free reflux from the gastrointestinal tract and these patients should be extubated when fully awake and sitting upright. Even the presence of a large double-lumen tube can cause a degree of laryngeal incompetence and therefore all patients fare better in a sitting position following thoracotomy. The upright position also favours more efficient respiration and diaphragmatic movement. Patients are sat up, therefore, following the removal of the endobronchial tube and allowed to breathe oxygen-enriched air. Further postoperative care is supervised in a high-dependency area or intensive care unit.

ENDOBRONCHIAL INTUBATION
AND ONE-LUNG ANAESTHESIA

Theoretical indications for endobronchial intubation range from the absolute to relative (Table 5.2). Isolation of the lungs is essential if there is severe bleeding or the presence of copious infected secretions in one of them. Endobronchial intubation is also mandatory to control ventilation and prevent the spread of secretions in the presence of a large bronchopleural fistula following pneumonectomy. Oesophageal surgery, and even some types of lung resection, could be regarded as relative indications for endobronchial intubation because they can be carried out using endotracheal anaesthesia. In practice, however, the ability to collapse the lung on the side of surgery is extremely useful for most thoracic procedures and the majority of surgeons would expect to have this facility. A double-lumen endobronchial tube also prevents soiling of the non-surgical lung with blood and pus. Patients with gross infective lung disease such as bronchiectasis and tuberculosis uncommonly present for surgery in the UK but many tumours block large bronchi causing a build-up of infection and even abscess formation distally (Figs 5.3 and 5.4). Manipulation of the tumour at operation releases this infected material and this can, potentially, soil the non-diseased lung. The use of a double-lumen tube prevents this type of disaster.

SELECTION AND USE OF
ENDOBRONCHIAL TUBES

Single-lumen endobronchial tubes and certain types of bronchial blocker are no longer manufactured. Double-lumen tubes are by far the most common endobronchial tubes now in use and can be employed in most circumstances

Table 5.2 Indications for endobronchial intubation

Absolute	Fistula or rupture of the tracheobronchial tree
	Lung transplantation
	Bronchoplastic surgery (e.g. sleeve resection)
	Massive haemorrhage or profuse secretions
	Lung cysts
	Lung resection } One-lung anaesthesia is used to facilitate surgery if satisfactory oxygenation can be maintained
	Oesophageal surgery
Relative	Pleurectomy

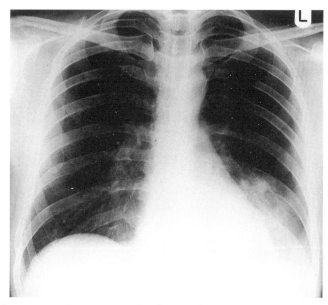

Fig. 5.3 Chest X-ray of a patient with left lower lobe pneumonia associated with a tumour blocking the left lower lobe.

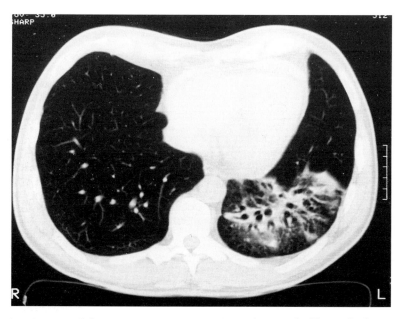

Fig. 5.4 CT scan of the same patient as in Fig. 5.3, showing build-up of infection and bronchiectasis distal to the tumour.

to separate the lungs and facilitate lung collapse. Some centres will have a large residual stock of single-lumen endobronchial tubes or may even adapt endotracheal tubes for a similar purpose. For completeness a brief discussion of the use of single-lumen tubes is set out below. Some readers may consider this to be of historical interest only! A short description of endobronchial intubation in infancy and the use of bronchial blockade in both adults and children is also included in this chapter.

Double-lumen endobronchial tubes

Double-lumen tubes are designed to provide independent channels for suction or ventilation to both lungs, and the lumen on one side is extended at an angle which favours its entry into one or other of the main bronchi. The other lumen terminates in the trachea, distal to the tracheal cuff, so that the non-intubated lung can also be ventilated. All makes of tube are manufactured on the same general pattern (Fig. 5.5) with oro-pharyngeal and bronchial curves (the distance between the two curves varying according to the diameter of the tube) and tracheal and bronchial cuffs. Right-sided tubes also incorporate a ventilation slot in the bronchial cuff in order to provide ventilation to the upper lobe bronchus, which arises much closer to the carina than on the left side. Despite overall similarities there are a number of differences in the detailed design and manufacture of double-lumen tubes currently available.

Double-lumen tubes are now available in disposable and non-disposable

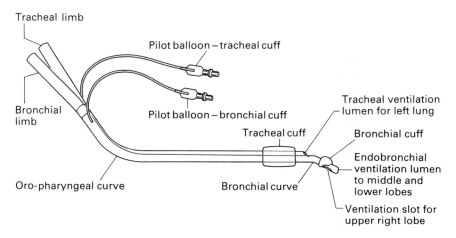

Fig. 5.5 Basic pattern of a modern right-sided double-lumen endobronchial tube.

forms. The disposable tubes have, understandably, begun to dominate the market and many types are now available (depending on country). In the UK the Bronchocath double-lumen tube (Mallinckrodt, Mallinckrodt Anesthesiology Division) appears to be the most widely used (Fig. 5.6) but a disposable, original-pattern, Robertshaw tube about to be marketed by Phoenix Medical (Leyland) Ltd is likely to be popular. A description of the Mallinckrodt tube and its practical application will illustrate the principles of using a disposable endobronchial tube. This tube will be compared, where relevant, with a similar, but not identical, product, the Rüsch disposable double-lumen tube (Fig. 5.7).

Despite the introduction of disposable tubes, rubber, non-disposable endobronchial tubes are still manufactured. Phoenix Medical (Leyland) Ltd now manufacture the original-pattern Robertshaw tube (Fig. 5.8) and a similar, but not identical, tube is manufactured by Rüsch (Fig. 5.9). Rüsch also continue to manufacture the Carlens' tube (or 'White' in right form) in the same soft rubber compound with a smooth coating of Silkolatex.

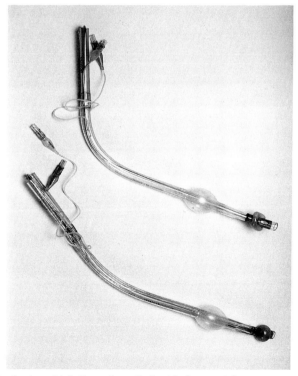

Fig. 5.6 Right (top) and left Bronchocath double-lumen tubes.

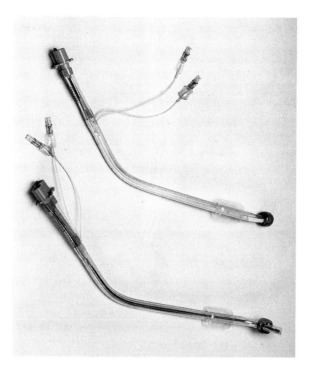

Fig. 5.7 Left (top) and right Rüsch disposable double-lumen tubes.

In British practice a double-lumen endobronchial tube is usually placed in the main bronchus of the lung contralateral to surgery when lung resection is planned. This allows the bronchial anastomoses to be fashioned in an unhurried manner with the tube in place. In some centres left-sided tubes are used exclusively to eliminate the problems associated with right upper lobe ventilation. If this is the case the tube must be withdrawn into the trachea before left pneumonectomy and left upper lobectomy are completed. This latter manoeuvre may allow the spread of secretions from lung to lung, despite the use of endobronchial suction. If a double-lumen tube is used for procedures other than lung resection, for example oesophageal surgery, it is eminently sensible to place a tube in the left main bronchus where the margin of safety is greatest.

Non-disposable double-lumen tubes

The original-pattern Robertshaw tube is now manufactured by Phoenix

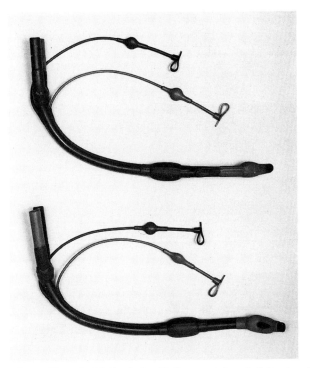

Fig. 5.8 Robertshaw, Phoenix Medical, double-lumen tubes (left (top) and right).

Medical Ltd in exactly the same dimensions as the Leymed version of the tube. The tube is made in right and left forms in three sizes: large, medium and small. Colour coding has recently been introduced in the manufacturing process to aid identification of various parts of the tube during manipulation and fibreoptic bronchoscopy. As a consequence of this the bronchial ventilation limb, the bronchial cuff and its pilot balloon are all made from blue rubber. The ventilation slot in the bronchial cuff of the original-pattern Robertshaw tube is particularly generous (Fig. 5.10a) and the work of McKenna *et al.* (1988) showed that this tube was much more likely to be opposite the right upper lobe orifice than a similar sized Bronchocath.

The Rüsch Robertshaw-type tube is made in right and left forms in sizes of 41, 37 and 35 Ch gauge (outside diameter) respectively. (Note: tube sizes are generally quoted as Charriere (Ch) gauge — equivalent to French gauge sizes.) The ventilation slot in the bronchial cuff of the right-sided tube is neither as wide nor as long as that of the original-pattern Robertshaw tube (Figs 5.10a and b) so the work of McKenna *et al.* does not apply to the Rüsch tube. However, further development of the Rüsch Robertshaw tube is planned for the near future.

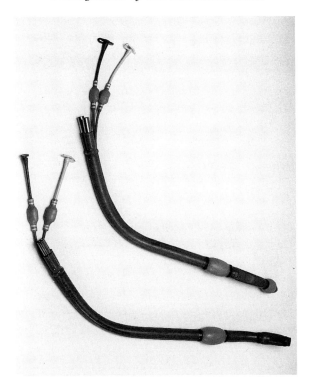

Fig. 5.9 Robertshaw, Rüsch, double-lumen tubes (left (top) and right).

The Carlens' and White tubes have a carinal hook which is designed to aid placement and stability within the bronchial tree (see Fig. 1.6). This hook is relatively difficult to advance through the larynx and can cause damage to the respiratory tract. These tubes are not widely used in the UK.

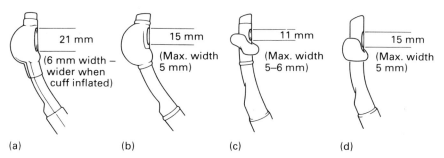

Fig. 5.10 (a) Upper lobe ventilation slot — Phoenix Medical Robertshaw tube; large, rubber. (b) Upper lobe ventilation slot — Rüsch Robertshaw tube; large 41 FG, rubber. (c) Upper lobe ventilation slot — Bronchocath (Mallinckrodt) disposable tube; 41 FG. (d) Upper lobe ventilation slot — Rüsch disposable tube; large 41 FG. Note: drawings not to scale.

Rubber tubes seem to move less *in situ* than disposable tubes but, in general, they are bulkier and less suitable for use in small patients. The rigidity of rubber tubes is also a disadvantage if it is necessary to advance the tube into position over a fibreoptic bronchoscope (see p. 96). The increase in laryngeal and mucosal damage previously attributed to rubber non-disposable tubes is not a significant clinical problem but, as with all endobronchial tubes, bronchial rupture can occur if the bronchial cuff is overinflated.

Disposable double-lumen tubes

The Bronchocath double-lumen tubes (Figs 5.6 and 5.10c) are made of polyvinylchloride in right and left forms in a wide range of sizes — 41, 39, 37 and 35 Ch gauge respectively. There is also a smaller 28 gauge tube made only in left form. The bronchial cuffs of the Bronchocath tube are colour coded in blue for easy identification during fibreoptic bronchoscopy and the configuration of the right bronchial cuff (Fig. 5.10c) is designed to improve efficiency of right upper lobe ventilation. This design feature has not been wholly successful, however. The tubes are relatively long and need to be placed carefully to avoid blocking off the upper lobe orifice both on the right and left sides. The tubes are presented with an indwelling metal stylet to stiffen the tube. This must be removed once the tube has been placed through the vocal cords before it is advanced into position.

The Rüsch disposable tubes (Figs 5.7 and 5.10d) are available in a wider range of sizes to the Bronchocath, as smaller 26 and 28 Ch gauge tubes are available in right and left forms. A range is also made incorporating a carinal hook. The internal diameter of the individual limbs of the Rüsch tubes is, however, significantly smaller than the comparable Bronchocath tubes. This is a distinct disadvantage as far as the use of the fibreoptic bronchoscope is concerned. The Olympus LF-1 anaesthetic fibreoptic bronchoscope/laryngoscope can be passed down a Bronchocath tube as small as 35 Ch gauge, for example, provided there are no irregularities in the internal plastic moulding. It is difficult to pass the same instrument down a 39 Ch gauge Rüsch disposable tube once it is *in situ*.

An original-pattern Robertshaw tube is soon to be introduced in a disposable form by Phoenix Medical Ltd. This will be made from a light rubber formulation but in other respects will be similar to the reusable type of tube.

Technique of placing double-lumen endobronchial tubes

A suitable double-lumen tube and its connections (Fig. 5.11) are selected and

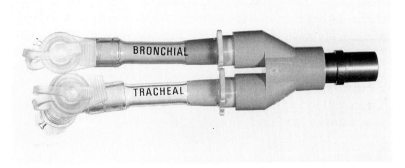

Fig. 5.11 Double-lumen tube connector.

checked. The author prefers to use either a medium or large, original-pattern, Robertshaw tube in patients of suitable size because they are stable in use and more likely, in the case of a right tube, to be opposite the right upper lobe orifice following blind placement. If intubation is likely to be difficult the more malleable plastic disposable tubes, such as the Bronchocath, seem to offer an advantage, and they are also indicated in the presence of infection and where long-term intubation is envisaged. The Bronchocath and Rüsch disposable tubes are also marketed in a wide range of sizes and are therefore more suitable for small female patients.

The size of tube chosen for an individual patient is somewhat empirical. Large tubes (corresponding to 41 and 39 Ch gauge) are usually selected in tall male adults and a medium tube (approximately 37 Ch gauge) is initially tried in the smaller male or taller female patient. The small Robertshaw tube is difficult to place optimally and as it will not allow the passage of the Olympus LF-1 bronchoscope it is preferable to use the 35 Ch gauge Bronchocath in small female patients.

Prior to endobronchial intubation laryngoscopy is carried out in the usual way. The double-lumen tube is turned through 90° so that the concavity of the endobronchial extension faces upwards and then it is advanced between the vocal cords. Once within the trachea any internal stylet is removed and the tube is turned back through 90° so that the endobronchial extension is likely to enter the appropriate bronchus as the tube is advanced 'blindly' towards the carina. If it is difficult to place the tube in the larynx (often because it is deflected by the teeth) a malleable bougie can be used to 'railroad' the tube into position through the vocal cords. In cases of extreme difficulty it may be necessary to use a fibreoptic bronchoscope from the outset.

If the double-lumen tube fails to advance or enters the wrong bronchus it is occasionally possible to redirect it once the patient's head has been rotated away from the side of required endobronchial intubation. This latter manoeuvre straightens the angle between the trachea and the bronchus to be intubated. If endobronchial intubation proves at all difficult, however, it is much quicker and safer to guide the tube into the appropriate bronchus with the fibreoptic bronchoscope.

Once the double-lumen tube is in place both the cuffs are inflated, taking particular care not to overdistend the bronchial cuff by inflating it just enough to achieve an airtight seal when ventilation is confined to that side. This can be simply checked by feeling for an air leak via the open tracheal limb of the tube. Both the tracheal and bronchial cuffs can remain inflated during surgery, and one-lung ventilation is achieved by clamping the appropriate limb of the catheter mount (Fig. 5.11) and opening the suction cap of that limb to allow the lung to deflate. This limb of the tube should be sucked out after surgery before ventilation is re-established.

The position of double-lumen tubes should be checked by alternate auscultation of both lung fields, paying particular attention to the left upper zone with a left tube and the area of the right upper lobe with a right tube. A great deal of information can also be gained from observing chest movement and feeling the change in manual inflation pressure as alternate lungs are ventilated. These checks are repeated after the patient has been positioned for thoracotomy. There is increasing evidence that clinical checks of this nature are inaccurate however, particularly with the relatively longer disposable tubes, and that it is preferable to check the position of endobronchial tubes with a fibreoptic bronchoscope.

Fibreoptic bronchoscopy
and the positioning of double-lumen tubes

Fibreoptic bronchoscopy can be used in three different ways to facilitate the accurate placement of double-lumen tubes. It can be used: (1) in a conventional manner to overcome a difficult laryngeal intubation; (2) to check and adjust the position of tubes previously placed 'blindly'; and (3) to 'railroad' double-lumen tubes into position using direct vision once they have been placed through the larynx.

The introduction of slim, relatively inexpensive, anaesthetic fibreoptic bronchoscopes/laryngoscopes such as the Olympus LF-1 has made the use of fibreoptic bronchoscopy a practical possibility in most centres. The Olympus LF-1 is a robust instrument that has a tip of 3.8 mm in diameter which can be passed down the lumen of endobronchial tubes as small as a 35 Ch gauge Bronchocath. Considerably smaller and more sophisticated paediatric bronchoscopes are now available but, although these instruments have superior optics, they are more expensive and probably too delicate for routine use during adult thoracic surgery.

Following auscultation fibreoptic bronchoscopy is used as a further, and more accurate, check of the position of a double-lumen tube. The broncho- scope is first passed down the tracheal limb of the double-lumen tube to check the position of the bronchial cuff. Ventilation is continued to the opposite lung and a careful check is kept on oxygenation by means of pulse oximetry. If the bronchoscope is a good fit in the suction cap of the catheter mount it may be feasible to continue ventilation to both lungs. With a left-sided double-lumen tube (Fig. 5.12) it is ascertained that there is a clear view down the right main bronchus and that the bronchial cuff is not obstructing the lower trachea or herniating over the carina. If the bronchial cuff of the tube is just visible below the carina in the left main bronchus (a blue colour-coded bronchial cuff is a distinct advantage in this situation) the tube is probably optimally placed. A second check is made by inspecting the endobronchial limb of the tube. With a left tube it is important to ensure that the distal portion of the tube is not blocking or impinging on the left upper lobe orifice (Fig. 5.12). It may be necessary to withdraw the tube slightly to avoid this situation and if this is the case it is mandatory to check the right tracheal limb again to ensure the bronchial cuff is not now obstructing this side. If this occurs a shorter tube is indicated.

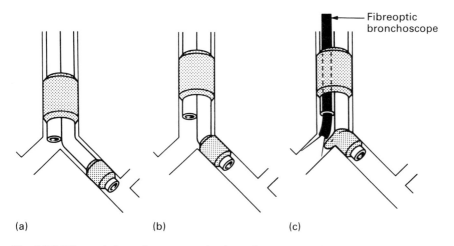

(a) (b) (c)

Fig. 5.12 Fibreoptic bronchoscopy — checking the position of a left-sided double- lumen tube. (a) Innermost acceptable position. (b) Outermost acceptable position. (c) Herniating cuff.

When a right-sided double-lumen tube is in place the tracheal limb is again checked first to ensure there is a clear view into the left main bronchus. It may be possible to identify a portion of the bronchial cuff just to the right of the carina but this provides little useful information, particularly with the bronchial cuff design of the Bronchocath. The crucial bronchoscopic check of a right-sided tube is down the endobronchial limb. It is first ascertained that the tube is not blocking the middle lobe bronchus and then attention is paid to the right upper lobe orifice. The ventilation slot in the bronchial cuff of the tube, or at least a significant proportion of it, should be opposite the right upper lobe orifice (Fig. 5.13). If this is not the case it will be necessary to manipulate the tube under direct vision or alternatively change the tube for one of a different size. If significant manipulation is used to position the ventilation slot so that there is a clear view of the trifurcation of the right upper lobe it is mandatory to check the tracheal limb again to ascertain that this remains clear. Unfortunately plastic disposable tubes are relatively 'springy' at body temperature and tend to move back into their original position if an excessive twist is put on them during manipulation. It is hardly surprising that problems with right upper lobe ventilation occur during surgery and that right upper lobe collapse is not uncommon following the use of a right-sided double-lumen tube.

It is advisable to repeat the above checking procedures after the patient has been positioned for surgery because, as previously mentioned, endobronchial tubes may move with flexion and extension of the neck. There is also no doubt that movement of tubes can occur during surgery. Plastic tubes appear more liable to move. They soften at body temperature, have a smooth

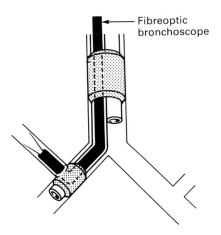

Fig. 5.13 Right-sided double-lumen tube in position.

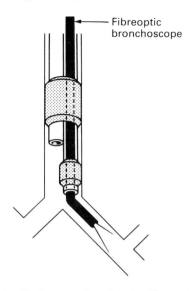

Fig. 5.14 Positioning a double-lumen tube with the fibreoptic bronchoscope.

surface and tend to be extruded from the main bronchus by the nature of their bronchial cuff inflation.

The above checking procedures should be used if there is any doubt about the position of a double-lumen tube, and some anaesthetists would consider this mandatory in all cases because of the inaccuracy of clinical checks.

One final use of the fibreoptic bronchoscope is in the initial placement of endobronchial tubes under direct vision. It is not always possible to site a double-lumen tube in the appropriate bronchus using a 'blind' placement technique even when the bronchial anatomy is normal. In these circumstances it is a relatively simple task to insert a double-lumen tube into the trachea, locate the appropriate main bronchus with a fibreoptic bronchoscope passed down the tube and then 'railroad' or slide the tube into position over the bronchoscope (Fig. 5.14). This technique is particularly useful in patients with distorted tracheobronchial anatomy (Fig. 5.15).

SINGLE-LUMEN ENDOBRONCHIAL TUBES

Although they are no longer manufactured we continue to use single-lumen endobronchial tubes in two specific, but rare, instances. Firstly, a single-lumen endobronchial tube is inserted in the lung opposite surgery when a pleuropneumonectomy is to be undertaken for a completely destroyed lung and, secondly, a similar tube may be useful when an anterior mediastinal

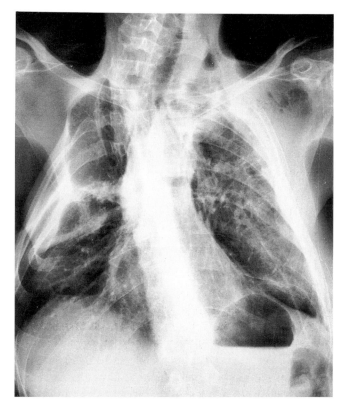

Fig. 5.15 Chest X-ray of a patient with extensive fibrous parenchymal disease. There is a previous thoracoplasty on the right and the patient was scheduled for left upper lobectomy and thoracoplasty. The fibreoptic bronchoscope was used to guide a right-sided Bronchocath double-lumen tube into position under direct vision.

tumour is compressing both the trachea and main bronchi. In the former situation the tracheobronchial anatomy is often distorted and it is essential to place a tube accurately in the lung opposite surgery. As the whole lung is to be removed surgically there is no requirement for the flexibility of two-lung ventilation provided by a double-lumen tube. In the latter case a single-lumen tube can be used to accurately negotiate a compressed airway and keep this open whilst tumour is resected (Chapter 10).

A Gordon–Green tube (Fig. 1.5) is used in the right main bronchus and a Brompton–Pallister tube in the left (Table 1.2). Both tubes are mounted on a Magill intubating bronchoscope and placed in the appropriate bronchus under direct vision. The optics of the narrow intubating bronchoscope are poor but it is easy to enhance the view by placing a modern optical telescope down the central lumen.

In the future we will probably use modern disposable double-lumen tubes, placed under direct vision with the fibreoptic bronchoscope, in the clinical situations described above. On the other hand it may be possible to use a long endotracheal tube for endobronchial intubation, provided that right upper lobe ventilation is not considered to be of vital importance.

ENDOBRONCHIAL INTUBATION IN INFANCY

Endobronchial intubation is rarely indicated in infants (see Chapter 7) but can be achieved satisfactorily using plain Portex endotracheal tubes which mould at body temperature to conform to the shape of the airway. The diameter chosen should be the same or one size smaller than would be used for endotracheal intubation, and the tube is cut so that its length is 1 cm greater than the distance from mouth to carina as measured on a lateral chest X-ray. The bevel is unaltered for left-sided endobronchial intubation but, for the right, a new and elongated bevel must be fashioned facing the opposite direction so that the right upper lobe is not obstructed. Once within the trachea, the tube is rotated through 180° so that the advancing tip will pass along the wall of the trachea on the side to be intubated. The head of the infant is pulled away from that side while the tube is advanced until the full length has been inserted. This displacement helps to guide the tip of the tube into the correct bronchus. Once in position it is rotated through a further 180° so that the longitudinal curve bears the usual relationship to the trachea and the terminal opening faces freely into the bronchus of the ventilated lung. Correct positioning of the tube is confirmed by auscultation.

THE USE OF ENDOBRONCHIAL BLOCKERS

Bronchial blockade is now rarely indicated in the developed world but can be useful for isolating single lobes in certain situations. For example, a bronchial blocker can be used to isolate a diseased left lower lobe from a normal upper lobe and lingula. We currently use Fogarty embolectomy catheters for this purpose in both adults and children.

After induction of anaesthesia and preliminary bronchoscopy, a Fogarty catheter of suitable size is chosen and placed through the patient's nose and then into the trachea using Magill's forceps and a laryngoscope. This route of insertion provides greater stability of the blocker once it is in place, particularly in children. The bronchoscope is then re-inserted into the trachea and the catheter manipulated into position under direct vision. Once in place the Fogarty balloon is inflated and the bronchoscope carefully withdrawn. An endotracheal tube, possibly one size smaller than normal, is then placed along side the catheter in the trachea and ventilation is continued. Care must be taken not to dislodge the catheter when the patient is turned into position for surgery. Great vigilance is also required in case the blocker becomes dislodged during surgery. If ventilation suddenly becomes difficult, with high inflation pressures, it is likely that the catheter has moved and the balloon is blocking a major airway. If this occurs it is essential that the balloon is rapidly deflated despite the risk of spreading infected secretions.

An alternative to the use of a Fogarty catheter in adults is the Univent tube which comprises an endotracheal tube with a moveable blocker attached. This device is not generally available in the UK but has achieved some popularity in North America. The tube comprises a tracheal tube with a small channel through the anterior internal wall which holds a blocker with a low pressure, high volume cuff. The tube is placed in the trachea in the usual way and the blocker advanced either blindly, or preferably under fibreoptic control, to block the appropriate lobe or segment. This tube can be used for the control of infected secretions or simply to provide one-lung anaesthesia.

FURTHER READING

Anaesthetic technique

See Further Reading section in Chapter 4.

Monitoring

Brodsky J.B., Shulman M.S., Swan M. & Mark J.B.D. (1985) Pulse oximetry during one-lung ventilation. *Anesthesiology*, **63**, 212–214.

Desiderio D.P., Wong G., Shah N.K., Liu J., Loughlin C.J. & Bedford R.F. (1990) A clinical evaluation of pulse oximetry during thoracic surgery. *Journal of Cardiothoracic Anesthesia*, **4**, 30–34.

Greeblott G.B., Tremper K.K., Barker S.J., Gerschultz S. & Gehrich J.L. (1991) Continuous blood gas monitoring with an intraarterial optode during one-lung anesthesia. *Journal of Cardiothoracic and Vascular Anesthesia*, **5**, 365–367.

Zaune U., Knarr C., Kroselmann M., Pauli M.F.H., Boeden G. & Martin E. (1990) Value and accuracy of dual oximetry during pulmonary resections. *Journal of Cardiothoracic Anesthesia*, **4**, 441–452.

Selection and use of endobronchial tubes

Benumof J.L. (1988) Improving the design and function of double-lumen tubes. Editorial. *Journal of Cardiothoracic Anesthesia*, **2**, 729–733.

Björk V.O. & Carlens E. (1950) The prevention of spread of secretions during pulmonary resection by the use of a double-lumen catheter. *Journal of Thoracic Surgery*, 20, 151–157.

Brodsky Jay B. & Mark J.B.D. (1991) Bilateral upper lobe obstruction from a single double-lumen tube. *Anesthesiology*, 74, 1163–1164.

Brodsky Jay B., Shulman M.S. & Mark J.B.D. (1985) Malposition of left-sided double-lumen endobronchial tubes. *Anesthesiology*, 62, 667–669.

Burton N.A., Watson D.C., Brodsky Jay B. & Mark J.B.D. (1983) Advantages of a new polyvinylchloride double-lumen tube in thoracic surgery. *The Annals of Thoracic Surgery*, 36, 78–84.

Clapham M.C.C. & Vaughan R.S. (1985) Bronchial intubation. A comparison between polyvinylchloride and red rubber double lumen tubes. *Anaesthesia*, 40, 1111–1114.

Conacher I.D. (1983) The urinary catheter as a bronchial blocker. *Anaesthesia*, 38, 475–477.

Conacher I.D. (1991) A coaxial technique for facilitating one-lung ventilation. *Anaesthesia*, 46, 400–403.

Foster J.M.G., Lau O.J. & Alimo E.B. (1983) Ruptured bronchus following endobronchial intubation. *British Journal of Anaesthesia*, 55, 687–688.

Ginsberg R.J. (1981) New technique for one-lung anesthesia using an endobronchial blocker. *Journal of Thoracic and Cardiovascular Surgery*, 82, 542–544.

Hanallah M. & Gomes M. (1989) Bronchial rupture associated with the use of a double-lumen tube in a small adult. *Anesthesiology*, 71, 457–459.

Hasan A., Low D.E., Ganado A.L., Norton R. & Watson D.C.T. (1992) Tracheal rupture with disposable polyvinylchloride double-lumen endotracheal tubes. *Journal of Cardiothoracic and Vascular Anesthesia*, 6, 208–211.

Holden M.P., Jones W.M., Bekassy S.M., Khan A. & Wooler G.H. (1972) Ruptured left main bronchus following right lung resection. *Anaesthesia*, 27, 204–208.

Inoue M., Shohtsu A. & Ogawa J. (1984) Endotracheal tube with moveable blocker to prevent intratracheal bleeding. *Annals of Thoracic Surgery*, 37, 497–499.

Kelley J.G., Gaba D.M. & Brodsky J.B. (1992) Bronchial cuff pressures of two tubes used in thoracic surgery. *Journal of Cardiothoracic and Vascular Anesthesia*, 6, 190–192.

Lack J.A. (1974) Endobronchial tube resistance. *British Journal of Anaesthesia*, 46, 461–462.

Lee K.G. & Phillips G. (1992) Red rubber Robertshaw tubes. *Anaesthesia*, 47, 545–546.

MacGillvray R.G. (1988) Evaluation of a new tracheal tube with a moveable bronchus blocker. *Anaesthesia*, 43, 25–26.

McKenna M.J., Wilson R.S. & Botelho R.J. (1988) Right upper lobe obstruction with right-sided double-lumen endobronchial tubes: a comparison of two tube types. *Journal of Cardiothoracic Anesthesia*, 2, 734–740.

Robertshaw F.L. (1962) Low resistance double-lumen endobronchial tubes. *British Journal of Anaesthesia*, 34, 576–579.

Saito S., Dohi S. & Naito H. (1985) Alteration of double-lumen position by flexion and extension of the neck. *Anesthesiology*, 62, 696–697.

Wagner D.L., Gammage G.W. & Wong M.C. (1985) Tracheal rupture following insertion of a disposable double-lumen tube. *Anesthesiology*, 62, 698–699.

Fibreoptic bronchoscopy and the positioning of double-lumen tubes

Brodsky Jay B. (1988) *Con*: Proper positioning of a double-lumen endobronchial tube can only be accomplished with endoscopy. *Journal of Cardiothoracic Anesthesia*, 2, 105–109.

Ehrenwerth J. (1988) *Pro*: Proper positioning of a double-lumen endobronchial tube can only be accomplished with endoscopy. *Journal of Cardiothoracic Anesthesia*, 2, 101–104.

Ovassapian A., Braunschweig R. & Joshi C.W. (1983) Endobronchial intubation using flexible fibreoptic bronchoscope. *Anesthesiology*, **59**, A501.

Shinnick J.P. & Freedman A.P. (1982) Bronchofiberscopic placement of a double-lumen endotracheal tube. *Critical Care Medicine*, **10**, 544–545.

Slinger P.D. (1989) Fibreoptic bronchoscopic positioning of double-lumen tubes. *Journal of Cardiothoracic Anesthesia*, **3**, 486–496.

Smith G.B., Hirsch N.P. & Ehrenwerth J. (1986) Placement of double-lumen endobronchial tubes. Correlation between clinical impressions and bronchoscopic findings. *British Journal of Anaesthesia*, **58**, 1317–1320.

Watson C.B. (1987) Fibreoptic bronchoscopy in thoracic anaesthesia. In: Gothard J.W.W. (ed.) *Thoracic Anaesthesia, Clinical Anaesthesiology*, Vol. 1, pp. 33–60. Baillière Tindall, London.

6: Postoperative Management and the Provision of Pain Relief

BEVERLY A. SUTTON

GENERAL PRINCIPLES

Thoracic surgery and anaesthesia inflict major respiratory and cardiovascular changes on the body which persist into the postoperative period for at least several days and often weeks. These changes are most exaggerated in the elderly, the obese, smokers and those with pre-existing cardiopulmonary disease. With advances in surgery and anaesthesia and the growing population of elderly, such patients form an increasing number of those presenting for thoracic surgery. The immediate postoperative care aims to avoid complications, and to detect the more incipient complications so that they can be treated promptly and effectively.

Recovery

Following major thoracic surgery patients who are not electively transferred to an intensive care unit should spend a period of time in a recovery area.

Here they can be closely monitored, initial investigations completed and adequate pain relief ensured. In addition the prompt attendance by an anaesthetist and/or surgeon is possible.

Most patients undergoing routine thoracotomy (e.g. lobectomy, pneumonectomy, pleurectomy) can usually be extubated at the end of surgery, either in the operating theatre or shortly after in the recovery room. Those undergoing more extensive surgery or in poor preoperative condition (poor nutritional state, extensive cardiovascular disease or cases of trauma), often benefit from a period of elective mechanical ventilation. This allows the patient to warm up, haemodynamic stability to be confirmed and the initiation of investigations. If there is any question as to whether immediate extubation is suitable, it is preferable to err on the side of caution, rather than attempt early extubation which if unsuccessful may result in the decline of the patient's condition and necessitate urgent intervention.

Initial investigations should include:

Full blood count
Serum electrolytes, urea and creatinine
Arterial blood gas analysis
Portable erect or semi-erect chest X-ray

Arterial blood gas analysis

Regular arterial blood gas sampling provides useful information on the patient's condition and progress. Interpretation of oxygen tension should always be in relation to the inspired oxygen concentration. For this reason the use of fixed-performance oxygen facemasks is preferable. Hypoxaemia and hypercarbia are both common following thoracic surgery, the mechanism of which is discussed further under altered lung mechanics. Mild acidosis is frequently seen, usually reflecting hypercarbia, but may have a metabolic element indicating decreased cardiac output and poor peripheral perfusion.

Chest X-ray

A chest X-ray should be performed in the erect or semi-erect position soon after surgery. Particular points to note are:
1 Position of mediastinum.
2 Full expansion of all lung fields, especially the right upper lobe if a right-sided double-lumen endobronchial tube has been used.

3   Evidence of pneumothorax. No significant pneumothorax should exist at this stage if full expansion of lung has been achieved at the end of surgery, and chest drains are patent.

4   Position of chest drains.

5   Position of endotracheal tube if present.

6   Position of internal jugular or subclavian venous lines.

7   Presence of any pleural fluid.

N.B. Check for pneumothorax if venous cannulation has been attempted on the non-operative side.

After a period in the recovery room, when the patient's condition is deemed to be satisfactory and adequate analgesia has been established, the patient can be transferred. A high-dependency ward provides the best setting for the management of these patients during the critical postoperative period, though such wards are not available in all surgical units. Wherever the patient is nursed it is essential that adequate monitoring facilities and sufficient nurses with experience in thoracic surgery are available.

Chest drainage

Selection and placement of chest drains

Chest drains must allow the escape of air or blood from the thorax and therefore wide-bore tubing is chosen to prevent obstruction by clot. Many surgeons prefer drainage tubes made of stiff plastic, which will not kink, and which contain lateral holes over a considerable length to aid drainage. A radio-opaque marker along the length of the tube aids the identification of drain position on the postoperative X-ray.

Two chest drains are commonly inserted following lung resection (other than pneumonectomy). Classically an apical drain is used to remove air which has risen towards the apex and a basal drain collects fluid which has gravitated downwards (Fig. 6.1a). An alternative, and equally effective approach, is to place anterior and posterior drains towards the apex with side-holes to provide basal drainage (Fig. 6.1b).

The underwater seal

The chest drains are joined to the outlet of an underwater seal drainage bottle (Fig. 6.2) as the pleural cavity is being closed. This prevents the lung collapsing again whilst the remaining layers of the chest wall are sutured,

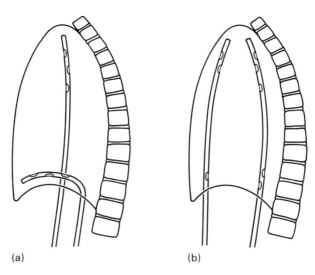

Fig. 6.1 (a) Apical and basal chest drains. (b) Anterior and posterior chest drains.

although intermittent positive pressure ventilation (IPPV) guards against this to a great extent. The underwater seal is merely a simple and reliable one-way valve which allows air to be expelled from the pleural space but not to enter during the next inspiration. In addition, the volume of blood or fluid drainage from the chest can be collected and measured accurately.

Various designs of drainage bottle are made but in theory a large diameter bottle is preferable with the chest drain terminating only 1–2 cm below the surface of the water. This provides minimal resistance to the escape of air but

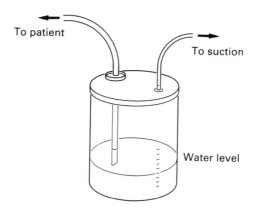

Fig. 6.2 An underwater seal chest drainage bottle.

a huge inspiratory effort would be needed to break the seal by drawing the water from the bottle into the chest. The drainage bottle should be well below the level of the patient's chest at all times. Elevation of the bottle results in ineffective drainage and the risk of the reservoir contents being siphoned into the chest. Clamping of the chest drains may be necessary during transfer of the patient. This can result in rapid accumulation of air in the pleural space resulting in a tension pneumothorax, particularly if there is a large air leak from the lung. If at all possible, therefore, drains should be left unclamped but below the patient during transfer. Inadvertent disconnection of chest drains will result in air entering the thorax from the atmosphere and collapse of the lung. Rapid reconnection of the drains and the re-establishment of suction resolves the situation.

The use of suction with chest drains

The space below the water in an underwater seal drain is vented to atmosphere through a short tube, although, more often, suction is applied here to facilitate drainage. Suction promotes expansion of the lung and assists the escape of air or fluid from the pleural space. It also eliminates the possibility of air entering the chest, because even the most vigorous inspiratory effort cannot overcome the negative pressure and so break the seal. Low pressure suction (approximately 5 kPa) is usually applied but this must be provided via a pump that is capable of clearing relatively large volumes of air. Modern pipeline low pressure suction units (Fig. 6.3) are usually sufficient to maintain a negative pressure in spite of all but the largest air leaks. Low pressure, low volume devices such as the Roberts pump merely act as an obstruction to drainage in this situation and may lead to collapse of the lung and surgical emphysema, particularly during coughing.

Removal of chest drains

Chest drains are removed when they have ceased to function. From the practical point of view this means when air or fluid loss has not occurred over the preceding 12–24 hours and when the pleural space has been obliterated by the formation of adhesions, as evidenced by the chest X-ray, the cessation of bubbling within the drainage bottle and the reduction of the respiratory swing of the water level. If there is no air leak, the fluid level will move gently in the drainage tubing during quiet spontaneous respiration but will cease to swing when the lung is fully expanded and opposed to the chest wall, or if the drain is blocked. Some surgeons prefer to clamp chest drains for a period

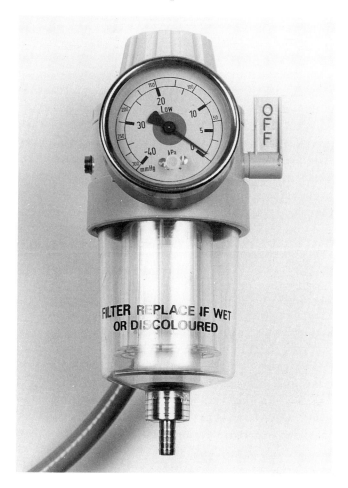

Fig. 6.3 Wall-mounted low pressure suction unit.

of 24 hours and then remove them if there is no evidence of air accumulation on chest X-ray. This approach is considered to be unnecessary and illogical by others.

Chest drains are removed by a competent trained nurse. There may be momentary discomfort during removal of chest drains and a natural tendency for patients to inspire. Removal is therefore undertaken during a Valsalva manoeuvre at full inspiration, thereby maintaining a positive intrapleural pressure and preventing influx of air. A purse-string suture placed around the chest drain at surgery is tightened as the drain is removed, to prevent air entering through the wound. A chest X-ray is taken immediately after this procedure to check that the lung remains fully inflated with no evidence of pneumothorax.

Chest drainage after pneumonectomy

Air leak does not occur after pneumonectomy and therefore chest drainage is not mandatory. Some surgeons, therefore, close the chest without a drain if they are confident that there is no significant bleeding. If a chest drain is not inserted, air is aspirated from the pneumonectomy space at the end of the operation, with the patient in the supine position. This can be done simply with a 50 ml syringe and three-way tap connected to a long intravenous cannula placed through the chest wall. Air is aspirated until there is a slight 'pull' on the syringe, indicating a negative pressure within the chest. At this stage the mediastinum, which will have migrated towards the dependent lung during lateral thoracotomy, should be approximately central or slightly towards the side of surgery. This position can be verified crudely by feeling the position of the trachea and more accurately by inspecting the post-operative chest X-ray. Occasionally it may be necessary to aspirate further air in the postoperative period.

Some surgeons prefer to place a chest drain in all pneumonectomy patients. This is usually a single basal drain (Fig. 6.4) which is left clamped but connected to an underwater seal drain. Traditionally the clamp is released for 2–3 minutes in every hour in order to reveal excessive blood loss and centralize the mediastinum by releasing trapped air. In spite of traditional teaching, however, a small number of surgeons leave the chest drain unclamped after pneumonectomy. This does not appear to cause excessive mediastinal shift but can lead to paradoxical mediastinal movement and less effective sputum clearance of the remaining lung.

Suction is *not* applied to a pneumonectomy drain under any circumstances. This will pull the mediastinum across and severely impede or totally obstruct venous return to the heart with disastrous consequences. Pneumonectomy drains are removed the day after surgery if there is no active bleeding. This allows the pneumonectomy space to fill with exudate and fluid in the usual manner (see Chapter 7).

Fluid balance

Intraoperative fluid and blood replacement will depend on the extent of surgical bleeding, preoperative hydration and haemoglobin. Postoperative intravenous fluid replacement is required for at least 24 hours and frequently

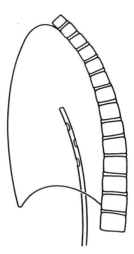

Fig. 6.4 Site of a basal pneumonectomy chest drain.

longer. Blood and exudate loss via the chest drains in the first 24 hours is usually of the order of 500–1000 ml. An immediate postoperative haemo-globin of less than 10 g/dl usually requires transfusion to prevent an unacceptably low haemoglobin developing.

Large amounts of plasma may be lost in the form of an exudate from the lung surface, pleura and chest wall. Such losses are not always obvious, and if not adequately replaced signs of hypovolaemia may develop. Personal experience in our department has shown that most patients require 1–2 ml/kg/h of a balanced crystalloid solution. However, all cases are individual and replacement should be balanced against the patient's clinical state, with particular attention to systemic and venous pressure and urinary output.

Occasionally, extensive intraoperative blood loss occurs necessitating massive blood transfusion. Postoperatively, attention should be paid to any coagulopathy, with transfusion of platelets, fresh frozen plasma and cryo-precipitate as necessary to correct any clotting defect.

Patients whose analgesia is controlled by means of epidural local anaes-thesia may experience extensive sympathetic block with vasodilatation and hypotension. Correction of such hypotension may require large volumes of intravenous fluid which is often poorly tolerated by the elderly, especially those with concomitant ischaemic heart disease. It is often preferable to control the hypotension by carefully titrated doses of a vasoconstrictor such as ephedrine. It is essential to differentiate between absolute hypovolaemia due to bleeding as opposed to the relative hypovolaemia associated with vasodilatation.

Many patients undergoing thoracic surgery do not need insertion of an indwelling urinary catheter, providing they have normal renal function, an uncomplicated postoperative course and experience no difficulty in micturition. However, it would seem prudent to insert a urinary catheter at the time of surgery in patients with evidence of pre-existing renal dysfunction, those undergoing extensive surgery or who give a history of prostatism. Unfortunately a significant number of patients receiving analgesia via the epidural route will experience postoperative urinary retention and require catheterization.

Dysrhythmias

Dysrhythmias are a well known complication of thoracic surgery, the incidence increasing with the age of the patient. Most occur in the first 3 days following surgery, the majority within the first 24 hours, with the highest proportion developing in the immediate perioperative period. Rhythm disturbances are a serious complication, associated with a significant mortality, especially following pneumonectomy.

Supraventricular tachydysrhythmias and atrial fibrillation in particular are the most common. There is evidence to suggest that they more frequently develop in those undergoing left thoracotomy, intrapericardial dissection and in patients with bronchogenic malignancy. Dysrhythmias are most common in patients with evidence of pre- or postoperative pulmonary oedema, suggesting a volume–pressure phenomenon.

Atrial fibrillation, atrial flutter and multifocal atrial tachycardia can be associated with a rapid ventricular response and haemodynamic collapse. Several aetiological factors have been identified; increased vagal activity, hypoxia, electrolyte and acid–base disturbance are regarded as the most important. The role and interaction of each remain unclear and they are by no means inevitable findings.

Prophylaxis

β-Blockers, calcium channel antagonists and digoxin have all been used to control the ventricular response. Digoxin has been used extensively for many decades, but its prophylactic value in preventing the emergence of tachydysrhythmias is questionable. Ritchie *et al.* (1990), in a prospective randomized trial, failed to find any advantage in the prophylactic use of digoxin in elective thoracic surgery. This contrasts with much previously reported work, but these older studies were predominantly retrospective and lacked sophisticated means of monitoring rhythm disturbances.

Borgeat *et al.* (1991) have shown that flecainide (Type 1C anti-arrhythmic) proved superior to digoxin in the prevention of post-thoracotomy tachy-dysrhythmias, and reported no adverse effects. More recently serious concern has been raised regarding the safety of flecainide. Flecainide was included in the Cardiac Arrhythmia Suppression Trial, (Echt *et al.*, 1991) a study designed to improve the long-term survival following myocardial infarction. Despite impressive efficacy, at 10 months follow-up the flecainide group had more than double the mortality of the placebo group. Comparable placebo-controlled trials have not been performed to determine if flecainide is associated with a higher risk of mortality in other patient groups. Until established one way or the other, the prophylactic use of flecainide in post-thoracotomy patients should proceed with the greatest care.

Management

First line management must be directed at correction of obvious aetiological factors such as hypoxaemia and hypokalaemia. Occasionally this is sufficient. More frequently though the patient fails to respond or no causal factor can be identified. In general most patients respond to digitalization, almost always reverting to sinus rhythm. Medication is usually continued for several weeks before withdrawal is attempted. Those patients with atrial fibrillation who remain refractory to digoxin or who show marked cardiovascular compromise invariably respond to direct current (DC) shock.

Alteration in respiratory mechanics following thoracic surgery

Operations on the chest produce clinically significant changes in ventilatory mechanics and pulmonary gas exchange.

Functional residual capacity

The most important alteration of lung volumes is the reduction in functional residual capacity (FRC) and its relationship to closing volume (CV). General anaesthesia reduces FRC by approximately 18% regardless of the technique or agents used. In addition, the effect of body posture is such that a change from sitting to supine is accompanied by a decrease of FRC of the order of 20%.

Closing volume

Elastic recoil of the lungs diminishes with age and the CV increases towards FRC. Smoking appears to have the same effect on CV as adding 10 years to one's age. By middle-age, CV may exceed FRC in the supine position and by the seventh decade CV may be greater than FRC even in the upright position. Both general anaesthesia and posture have minimal effect on CV.

When CV exceeds FRC, airway closure occurs during tidal breathing and atelectasis develops in the dependent lung segments. Hypoxaemia results from the venous admixture caused by regional ventilation/perfusion mismatch and by shunting of pulmonary capillary blood through closed alveoli. Factors which further exacerbate the effects of airway closure are the volumes of tracheobronchial secretions, and the patient's ability to clear these. Patients with copious secretions who are unwilling or unable to cough forcefully will have a greater tendency for airway closure and alveolar collapse.

Chronic obstructive pulmonary disease

Chronic obstructive pulmonary disease (COPD) is a frequent finding in patients presenting for thoracic surgery. Such patients have abnormal mechanical lung function, ventilation disturbance and gas mixing. Because of the primary disease the residual volume and FRC are abnormally raised, and to a small degree protect from alveolar collapse postoperatively. Unfortunately the diseased alveoli are difficult to ventilate, even with maximum effort, and minute ventilation must be higher than normal to achieve adequate carbon dioxide clearance. Postoperative respiratory depression in these patients does not usually result in atelectasis, as would occur in normal lungs, but in carbon dioxide retention and hypoxaemia secondary to alveolar hypoventilation.

Postoperative ventilatory pattern

Following thoracic surgery there is restricted ventilation and an altered pattern of breathing (Fig. 6.5, Table 6.1). The characteristic mechanical abnormality is a reduction in vital capacity, tidal volume and forced expiratory volume, as well as FRC. The pattern of ventilation changes to monotonous shallow breathing without spontaneous deep breaths. The frequency of respiration increases with relative shortening of the inspiratory phase. Pain is the principal inhibitor of chest wall movement, but obesity, a supine position and interstitial oedema of damaged tissue all have a restrictive effect on ventilation. Postoperative hypoxaemia is almost always inevitable following thoracic surgery, and it is out of proportion to the actual quantity of lung removed or collapsed. Entwistle *et al.* (1991) have shown that 80% of patients exhibited a degree of hypoxaemia during the night

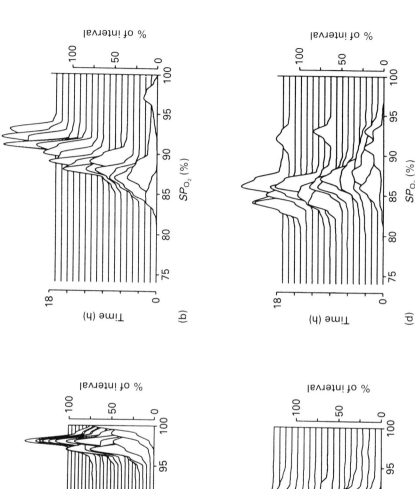

Fig. 6.5 (*see legend on facing page*)

Table 6.1 Numbers of patients (out of 20) showing a particular oxygen saturation pattern on the preoperative night and the first, second and fourth nights following thoracotomy (Entwistle *et al.*, 1991)

Oxygen saturation pattern	Night			
	Pre-op	1st	2nd	4th
Stable, not hypoxaemic	11	2	3	5
Stable, hypoxaemic but improving	0	8	0	0
Stable, hypoxaemic	9	5	12	11
Unstable, hypoxaemic	0	5	5	0

Note: the patients who were hypoxaemic before surgery, not surprisingly, remained so postoperatively

following surgery, with more than 50% of patients remaining hypoxaemic as late as the fourth postoperative night. Patients fell into four distinct groups: (1) not hypoxaemic; (2) stable, hypoxaemic but improving; (3) stable, constant hypoxaemia; (4) unstable, hypoxaemic and deteriorating. Not surprisingly patients who were hypoxaemic before surgery remained so following surgery. More interestingly, postoperative hypoxaemia could be predicted in only 50% of cases.

To minimize hypoxaemia and pulmonary complications postoperatively the following measures should be adopted:

Fig. 6.5 (*see facing page*) Patterns of oxygenation after thoracotomy. *Explanatory note:* The authors continuously measured oxygen saturation in a number of patients following thoracotomy. Recordings of saturation were taken by means of a computer every 15 seconds so that 240 samples were taken every 60 minutes. Compressed oxygen saturation distribution diagrams were plotted for each study period. Each curve represents a data collection interval of 1 hour and the height of the curve at each saturation value represents the percentage of the hour spent at that saturation. Patterns of tall, well-superimposed peaks were classed as stable. Patterns of flat peaks with much variation from hour to hour were classed as unstable. The authors identified four patterns of oxygen saturation distribution after operation:
(a) Stable, not hypoxaemic; normal oxygen saturation with narrow superimposed peaks indicative of good ventilatory control. (b) Stable, hypoxaemic but improving. The low oxygen saturation with broad peaks immediately after thoracotomy implies venous admixture as a result of atelectasis, in addition to impaired respiratory control. (c) Stable, hypoxaemic. Hypoxaemia caused by ventilation/perfusion mismatch, with good ventilatory control. (d) Unstable, hypoxaemic. Abnormal control and increased venous admixture throughout the period of monitoring. The numbers of patients in each group at different times in the postoperative period are shown in Table 6.1 (Entwistle *et al.*, 1991).

1   A provision of adequate analgesia without respiratory depression or excessive sedation.
2   An erect or semi-recumbent position so as to increase FRC.
3   Humidified oxygen to reduce tenacity of secretions.
4   Continuous oxygen therapy for at least the first four postoperative nights.
5   Regular physiotherapy.

Physiotherapy

The aim of physiotherapy is to reduce the incidence of postoperative complications, particularly pulmonary. Therapy commences preoperatively with optimizing of the patient's condition, especially with regard to pulmonary function. Patients need to be instructed in deep breathing exercises, diaphragmatic breathing, arm exercises and means to produce effective coughing whilst minimizing pain. In addition they need a realistic account of what to expect and to understand the importance of physiotherapy.

Therapy is based on rapid mobilization in addition to breathing exercises. Patients should be encouraged to undertake the various exercises regularly throughout the day, not merely when attended by the physiotherapist. As previously mentioned, adequate analgesia without excessive sedation is an essential component of postoperative management, if patients are to be able to comply with vigorous therapy.

Principles of treatment

Pulmonary complications are a major cause of morbidity following thoracic surgery. The incidence varies widely between published work depending on the criteria used. The reduced FRC is the single most important mechanical change, with alteration in pulmonary mechanics and respiratory control being secondary though important interacting factors. The maintenance or restoration of FRC is the key therapeutic goal. Techniques which encourage or force the patient to inspire deeply are the most clinically important. The aim is to interrupt the monotonous shallow restrictive pattern of breathing with intermittently sustained increases in transpulmonary pressure, in distension of the lung, and in lung volumes. Older techniques which encourage exhalation are deflationary and do not produce the desired increase in lung volumes. Measurement of vital capacity, which involves exhalation to residual volume, is included amongst these.

Additional techniques

Devices which have been used in an attempt to increase FRC include continuous positive airway pressure (CPAP), intermittent self-administered positive expiratory pressure ventilation (S-PEP) and incentive spirometry. Although attractive in theory the evidence that any of these can decrease the incidence of pulmonary complications is inconclusive. Frolund and Madsen (1986) found no benefit in the use of S-PEP following thoracotomy, when used in addition to conventional physiotherapy, either in terms of oxygenation or development of atelectasis. This confirms earlier work by Paul and Downs (1981), who also investigated the use of CPAP, and concluded that CPAP was the only method which reduced postoperative complications. Pinilla *et al.* (1990) found similar results with CPAP, but only in terms of improved oxygenation, the incidence of atelectasis was unaltered. It must be noted that CPAP only appears beneficial during its use, and a sustained effect after discontinuation was not seen. This would necessitate its employment for 24 hours or longer which raises problems of patient acceptability and interruption of sleep.

Craven *et al.* (1974) investigated the use of incentive spirometry in patients following upper abdominal surgery and found a significant reduction in the rate of pulmonary complications. They also noted that the subgroup which did best was the high-risk group (chronic respiratory disease and smokers). However, the value of incentive spirometry has not been confirmed by others.

Physiotherapy is an essential element in postoperative care following thoracotomy. The aim of all manoeuvres is to increase lung volumes, encourage clearance of secretions and allow rapid mobilization. The insertion of a mini-tracheostomy, either at the time of surgery or postoperatively, can greatly facilitate the removal of secretions by gentle suction. This is particularly useful in those with profuse bronchial secretions, those who exhibit difficulty in clearance of secretions and in the especially frail patient. Whether other techniques in addition to conventional therapy are of any benefit is still unclear, and further evaluation is needed.

POSTOPERATIVE ANALGESIA

Pain following thoracotomy is considered to be amongst the most severe that can be experienced postoperatively, and has been described by Loan and Morrison (1967) as near the top of iatrogenic causes. The intensity of pain invariably leads to heavy consumption of analgesics. Until recently postoperative pain has received inadequate attention. Donovan *et al.* (1987), in a randomly selected group of hospital patients, found that 58% experienced 'excruciating' pain at some time. In addition the working party for The Royal College of Surgeons of England and The College of Anaesthetists reporting on

'Pain After Surgery' (1990) concluded that treatment of pain '...has been inadequate and not advanced significantly for many years...'. Merely prescribing analgesia is ineffective as Donovan *et al.* noted, with less than a quarter of the amount ordered being given over a 24 hour period.

Relief of pain is not merely a humane gesture. Numerous reports exist of improved outcome with less postoperative complications in patients whose analgesia was adequate. This is particularly so in post-thoracic surgery where good pain relief has been repeatedly shown to improve pulmonary function and reduce the length of stay in hospital.

Source of pain

The skin incision begins at the level of T_2 or T_3 and extends downwards over the next seven or so dermatomes. The muscles latissimus dorsi, serratus anterior, pectoralis major and the intercostal muscles are either cut or retracted. The ribs are spread by use of retractors and the periosteum stripped. Intercostal nerves may be damaged at this stage or later when sutures are passed around the ribs to facilitate closure. During surgery the shoulder is extended and finally one or two large-bore drains are inserted through separate incisions.

All these structures are richly innervated. Following surgery noxious stimuli are conducted centrally via the following pathways:

from the chest wall and most of the pleura via the intercostal nerves;

from the diaphragmatic pleura via the phrenic nerve;

from the lung and mediastinal pleura via the vagus;

from the shoulder joint via spinal nerves C5–7;

the sympathetic nerves conduct pain of visceral origin, but their role is ill-defined.

It can be seen that the pain following thoracotomy originates from a wide area. Analgesia following chest surgery has attracted much clinical interest over the years and is well represented in the medical literature. In fact few operations seem to command so much attention. This is probably a reflection of the facts that the pain is amenable to such a wide variety of techniques and the benefits of good pain relief have significantly measurable effects in terms of morbidity.

New concepts in pain

Ideas and attitudes towards pain are changing. Increasing evidence suggests that the manner in which pain is treated has long-term implications extending beyond the immediate postoperative period.

The concept of the nervous system being a 'hard wired, line labelled system' now appears simplistic. Mounting research implies that the nervous system is capable of plasticity, with alterations in both structure and function as a result of previous experience, including trauma. The changes within the nervous system result in alteration in the way information from the periphery is handled, and are responsible for the generation of clinical pain.

Experimental work has demonstrated changes resulting in: peripheral sensitization of primary afferents; and central sensitization of dorsal horn neurones. After peripheral tissue injury the threshold for eliciting pain decreases, both within the area of injury and in the surrounding area. The pain is perceived over a greater area than one might anatomically suppose.

Central sensitization occurs in the spinal cord as a result of repeated identical stimuli evoking successively larger and larger responses, a phenomenon known as 'wind-up'. Changes in the dorsal horn ultimately result in altered perception of peripheral stimuli, which includes feeling pain in response to innocuous stimuli. In addition changes in the dorsal horn neurones alter the activity of preganglionic sympathetic fibres. Sympathetic fibres are capable of influencing primary sensory afferents, increasing their sensitivity to adrenergic stimuli, thus establishing a positive feedback circuit.

Clinical significance

In the management of pain the aim must be to reduce both the peripheral sensitization of primary afferents and the afferent-induced changes in central neurones, thus preventing the occurrence of plasticity.

The mechanism responsible for changes in primary afferents is complex and not fully understood. Substances such as histamine, bradykinin, substance P, the leukotrienes and prostaglandins are all present in damaged tissue. All have the ability to excite nociceptors or increase their sensitivity. At present the only clinical manoeuvre available to us to reduce the effect of these substances is with the non-steroidal anti-inflammatory group of drugs.

Central changes in the dorsal horn neurones appear to be more amenable to manipulation. Both opioids and local anaesthetics are capable of reducing these changes. Experimental evidence has shown that the dose of morphine necessary to prevent C-fibre-induced changes in the spinal cord is less than that required to suppress these changes once they have occurred.

Most of the work in this area has been laboratory-based animal experimentation and no reliable prospective human studies have as yet been published. Clinical impression has long been that pain is more easily and effectively treated if analgesia is administered before the onset of noxious stimuli. This has given rise to the concept of pre-emptive analgesia.

The results of prospective clinical studies in this area are eagerly awaited. It is hoped that pre-emptive analgesia will not only reduce early postoperative pain, but will also have a beneficial influence on the development of chronic postoperative pain.

Chronic post-thoracotomy pain

Long-term chronic pain following thoracotomy is being increasingly recognized. Most of the research into this problem has been retrospective, with no prospective studies as yet published. The nature, severity and duration of the pain vary considerably, and as an entity chronic post-thoracotomy pain encompasses a wide range of symptoms. No single definition of this condition presently exists. Most practitioners consider the presence of pain or altered sensation in or adjacent to the scar, which has persisted for more than 6 months and which is not related to persistent underlying pathology, as constituting the main features of the condition. The pain may be dull, burning or stabbing. Sensation may be altered from painful numbness to hyperaesthesia. Secondary features of back pain and frozen shoulder are often present.

The reported incidence of chronic post-thoracotomy pain ranges from 44–67%. In many the pain is mild and little affects daily living. Unfortunately there is a small but significant proportion of patients who develop pain of such severity as to seek further help in chronic pain clinics. From the available studies it appears that about 5% of all thoracotomy patients will develop severe, disabling, chronic pain.

The aetiology of chronic post-thoracotomy pain is unknown. There is evidence to suggest that patients who experience severe pain in the first 48 hours following surgery and those with high analgesic requirements are more likely to develop chronic pain. Aetiology is likely to be multifactorial, relating to surgical technique, perioperative analgesia and its efficacy, underlying pathology and individual patient psychology.

It has been suggested that cryoanalgesia may play a contributory part in the development of this syndrome. Roxburgh *et al.* (1987), Muller *et al.* (1989) and Conacher *et al.* (1986) all independently found evidence to suggest that long-term complications of neuralgia occurred with sufficient frequency to conclude that cryoanalgesia had no demonstrable role in the control of acute post-thoracotomy pain. In response to such concerns, Johannesen *et al.* (1990) examined a small group of patients where cryoanalgesia had been used. They found that 50% of the group had some hypoaesthesia associated with the scar, one patient had developed chronic pain, but there were no reports of hyperaesthesia. No definite evidence exists of a causal relationship between cryoanalgesia and chronic post-thoracotomy pain. As such pain develops in individuals who have not received cryoanalgesia, it alone cannot be responsible for the development of chronic pain, though it may well be contributory in some patients. It is interesting to note that cryotherapy has been used to treat post-thoracotomy neuralgia. Conacher (1986) treated 14 patients in this manner. Although a proportion of the patients gained some relief, a third felt that their symptoms were exacerbated.

Chronic post-thoracotomy pain is a serious condition and not easily treated. It has financial implications to the patient, the state and health resources. Long-term prospective follow-up of patients, examining the probable multifactorial nature of the condition, is urgently needed.

REGIONAL ANALGESIA

Intercostal nerve block

Intercostal nerve (ICN) blockade with local anaesthesia has been used extensively in the past to provide pain relief following thoracotomy. For a while its popularity fell, probably due to increasing use of epidural analgesia. More recently, interest has focused on ICN block with the introduction of variously sited catheters.

Technique

Each nerve is blocked by a separate injection and it is generally possible to block from T_2 to T_{11} or T_{12}. In order to block the lateral cutaneous branch it is necessary to inject the local anaesthetic posterior to its origin, at approximately the level of the mid-axillary line. The most commonly used surface landmark is the angle of the rib, which is easily palpable in all but the most obese subjects, and is readily accessible at the end of surgery whilst the patient remains in the lateral position.

Advantages

ICN block is simple to perform and in competent hands provides reliable anaesthesia over the distribution of injected nerves. It is not associated with sympathetic blockade and requires less intensive monitoring postoperatively than many other techniques. Although ICN block carries a risk of pneumothorax, this is not a consideration following thoracotomy providing a chest drain is inserted at the end of surgery.

Disadvantages

ICN block will not affect pain arising from the dome of the pleura, areas supplied by the posterior primary rami or conducted via the phrenic and vagus nerve. Consequently, as the sole form of analgesia it fails to provide adequate postoperative pain relief in most patients. Supplementary analgesia, usually in the form of opoids, is invariably required.

Local anaesthetics and duration of action

Between 3–5 ml of local anaesthetic is injected at each site. All commonly available agents have been used, but bupivacaine is generally favoured due to its longer duration of action. Unfortunately even with longer-lasting local anaesthetics the block is relatively short, lasting between 4 and 8 hours, although a prolonged effect is occasionally seen. This short duration of block limits the usefulness of ICN block, as repeated injections are not always practical.

A very real risk with ICN block is that of systemic toxicity. Large volumes of local anaesthetic are deposited in close proximity to the neurovascular bundle, systemic absorption readily occurs and high plasma concentrations are rapidly achieved. Various attempts have been made to increase the duration of action and limit systemic absorption. These have included addition of adrenalin, alkalinization and carbonation of local anaesthetics. Generally little useful impression is made on duration of action, though adrenalin does significantly reduce the peak serum concentration. The systemic effect of adrenalin also needs to be considered. Injecting 40 ml of commercially prepared bupivacaine with 1 in 200 000 adrenalin results in a total dose of 0.20 mg adrenalin.

Intercostal catheters

Further attempts to provide a more prolonged period of analgesia have involved the introduction of catheters. One or more catheters are introduced by the surgeon percutaneously into the intercostal space and parallel to the neurovascular bundle. The tip of the catheter is placed dorsal to the posterior axillary line and its position is checked manually and/or visually.

Safran *et al.* (1990) reported the use of a single catheter inserted immediately before the incision. A bolus injection was followed by a continuous infusion of lidocaine 1% at a rate of 1 mg/kg/h for 54 hours. No patient required additional analgesia during this period. Pharmacokinetic data obtained on a sample of patients showed both peak and steady-state serum concentrations to be below toxic levels. They did comment though that additional boluses may well have elevated serum levels to within the toxic range.

Kolvenbach *et al.* (1989) have investigated the use of three catheters; one in the incisional space, the others in the space immediately above and below. Analgesia was afforded by intermittent boluses of 0.5% bupivacaine, with an average daily dose of 330 mg. This regimen did not appear to provide such good analgesia, with a higher proportion of their control group reporting satisfactory pain relief compared to their study group. In addition they noted an increased incidence of tachydysrhythmias in the study group, although serum concentrations of bupivacaine remained below those associated with cardiotoxicity.

The introduction of catheters into the intercostal space has added a new dimension to an old technique, overcoming many of the previous disadvantages. The optimum number, position of catheter and choice of local anaesthetic are not yet established. Whether complications relating to systemic toxicity will limit further development has yet to be seen.

Extrapleural analgesia

As an extension of the intercostal space catheter technique, and in an attempt to extend the area of analgesia, various workers have been looking at extrapleural catheter placement.

Technique

An area of parietal pleura is retracted medially, starting at the posterior wound edge and extending to the vertebral bodies and two intercostal spaces above and below. A cannula is then introduced percutaneously and positioned to lie against the costovertebral joint, within the pocket formed by the retracted pleura. The parietal pleura is then simply attached to the posterior wound edge. Although the technique depends on an intact pleura, the method has been used in patients undergoing pleurectomy. The pleurectomy is performed in the usual manner except one area of the parietal pleura extending from the angle of the rib to the vertebral bodies at the level of the incision is left intact. The catheter is then carefully introduced into this isolated pocket.

Mode of action

Extrapleural blocks appear to differ from ICN blocks in that spread of local anaesthetic extends into the paravertebral space. Not only are local inter-costal nerves affected but the spread of local anaesthetic within adjacent paravertebral spaces results in a more extensive block which includes the posterior primary rami. One would therefore anticipate improved analgesia and the possibility of sympathetic blockade.

Sabanathan *et al.* (1990), in two separate studies using continuous extrapleural analgesia block, showed the bupivacaine study group had lower pain scores, required less supplementary opioid analgesia and had better preserved pulmonary function than the control group. All the differences were highly significant and very impressive. Additionally they recorded no com-plications of the technique and interestingly no evidence of sympathetic blockade.

Extrapleural analgesia adds between 10 and 20 minutes to the operating time, comparable with that required for extradural cannulation, appears highly efficacious in terms of analgesia and preservation of pulmonary function, and to date appears to be a safe technique.

Intrapleural analgesia

Instillation of local anaesthetics intrapleurally (that is between the visceral and parietal pleura) was first reported for the treatment of postoperative pain following cholecystectomy, renal and breast surgery. Promising results stimulated interest in its use for post-thoracotomy pain given the accessibility of the pleural space and ease of insertion of catheters.

Technique and mode of action

One or more catheters are introduced percutaneously by the surgeon before closure of the chest. The catheters are placed either against the posterior parietal pleura or more laterally in the posterior mid-clavicular line, at the level of the second or third intercostal space. Usually the catheter is loosely sutured in place.

The mode of action of intrapleural local anaesthetics is presumed to be due to diffusion through parietal pleura and intercostalis intimus muscle to have its effect on intercostal nerves. Whether diffusion to the paravertebral space occurs is uncertain, but is probably a variable and unpredictable feature. Investigators have found conflicting results in its efficacy. Factors which may prevent adequate analgesia are loss of local anaesthetic via the chest drains, dilution with residual irrigation fluid and/or blood, binding to blood proteins in the presence of haemothorax and rapid absorption from injured pleura and lung tissue.

Ferrante *et al.* (1991) found that between 30–40% of the administered dose was lost into the chest drains over a 4 hour period. The extent of such losses is unpredictable, and makes for difficulty in calculating drug dosage and further management in the face of analgesic failure.

Efforts to reduce these problems have involved placing the patient in a supine position and clamping of chest drains for 5–10 minutes after bolus injection. Neither of these techniques can be considered desirable practices in the early postoperative period. Use of more than one catheter appears to improve pain relief, but the addition of adrenalin makes no difference to the quality of analgesia, although it does reduce the peak serum concentration of local anaesthetic.

Although intrapleural analgesia appears a useful technique in some hands, and reduces opioid analgesia requirements, it is subject to so many variables that analgesia is unpredictable. Intrapleural analgesia is quick and simple to perform, but the results of the time taken to secure extrapleural access would appear to provide superior results.

Paravertebral block

The paravertebral space is the area the spinal nerve enters immediately after leaving the intervertebral foramen. The nerve divides into the anterior and posterior primary rami within the space and the sympathetic chain lies in the anterior aspect. Injection of local anaesthetic into the paravertebral space can produce a motor, sensory and sympathetic block, and provide localized unilateral segmental anaesthesia.

The identification of the paravertebral space is most easily achieved by a loss of resistance to injection as the needle passes through the costotransverse ligament. Both single shot injections and placement of a catheter are possible. Accidental puncture of the dura and pleura can occur and catheters can inadvertently be placed intrathecally, extradurally or intrapleurally. Limiting the length of catheter left in the space reduces the risk of misplacement, but increases the risk of the catheter being dislocated.

Although there is no direct communication between adjacent paravertebral spaces, injected solutions may spread via the loose connective tissue in each space. Purcell-Jones *et al.* (1987) have shown that injections within the paravertebral space are subject to variable spread. They demonstrated that in only 10% of cases was the injectate confined to the paravertebral space. In most cases the solution extends to the epidural space, and may on occasions spread bilaterally over 12 segments. Pleural spread was also occasionally seen. This conflicts with much clinical evidence which fails to demonstrate any contralateral spread.

As a regional technique paravertebral block has much to commend itself in the management of post-thoracotomy pain. Correct placement of local anaesthetic provides good analgesia over the chest wall including that supplied by the posterior primary rami. The possibility of unilateral sympathetic block reduces the risk of hypotension, bradycardia and urinary retention compared to extradural block. The risk of extension of the block, however, requires as vigilant observation postoperatively as if extradural block had been performed.

The increasing interest in extrapleural analgesia may result in blind percutaneous cannulation of the paravertebral space being superseded by direct visual placement of the extrapleural catheters by surgeons. However one distinct advantage of the paravertebral approach is that a sensory block can be established prior to the onset of surgical trauma, a factor which may have long-term significance.

Epidural local anaesthetics

Epidural local anaesthetics can provide excellent analgesia both intra- and postoperatively. Originally confined to obstetric anaesthesia, the technique has rapidly expanded into other surgical fields, including cardiothoracic anaesthesia.

To provide adequate analgesia for thoracic surgery with local anaesthetics a minimum sensory level of T_3–T_4 is required. To achieve this level requires considerable volume to be injected, especially if a lumbar approach is used. Positioning the patient horizontal with the operative side dependent can reduce the total volume required and produce localized unilateral block. Unfortunately change to a supine or semi-recumbent position produces a more extensive and bilateral block.

Lignocaine and bupivacaine remain the two most widely used agents, with bupivacaine generally favoured for its longer duration of action. Lignocaine has a more rapid onset, which may be useful when commenced preoperatively with the aim of establishing a certain level of sensory block prior to the onset of surgical stimuli. Lignocaine has anti-arrhythmic action, whilst bupivacaine is known to be prorhythmogenic. High serum concentrations of bupivacaine, especially rapidly rising, as may be seen after bolus injection, may add to the incidence of perioperative dysrhythmias in this vulnerable group.

Various attempts have been made to enhance the intensity of analgesia, thereby reducing the total dose of local anaesthetic used and limiting unwanted side effects. These have included a thoracic approach to the epidural space, addition of vasoconstrictors, alkalinization and carbonation of the local anaesthetics and, more recently, combination with opioids. The addition of opioids is becoming more popular with increasing recognition of their synergistic action enhancing analgesia with fewer adverse effects.

There are several disadvantages to the sole use of epidural local anaesthetics. The main problem lies in the height of the block required and its cardiovascular effects. Wattwill *et al.* (1985) using healthy volunteers, in the supine position, injected 5 ml of 0.5% bupivacaine via a thoracic epidural. They demonstrated a decrease in cardiac output by 33%, stroke volume by 22%, heart rate by 15% and systolic pressure by 5%. Given that the volume of local anaesthetic was considerably less than required for post-thoracotomy analgesia, and that their volunteers were healthy, one can predict severe cardiovascular compromise in patients who are generally older and frequently have coexisting ischaemic heart disease. The combination of high sympathetic block, cardiac depressant general anaesthetics and surgical blood loss can on occasions lead to cardiovascular collapse intraoperatively.

Other problems which occur with extensive regional block include symptoms of systemic toxicity, inhibited forceful coughing due to bilateral paresis of abdominal and intercostal muscles, urinary retention and motor block reducing mobility and increasing the risk of pressure sores.

Epidural local anaesthetics are useful to provide intraoperative analgesia, which may reduce the severity of subsequent pain. Their continued use as the sole method of analgesia into the postoperative period is limited by the high incidence of cardiovascular complications.

OPIOID ANALGESIA

Parenteral opioids

Intramuscular opioids were once the mainstay of all postoperative analgesia. They are rarely used today as the sole means of pain relief following thoracotomy. The disadvantages are ineffective pain relief with periods of distressing pain, punctuated by periods of excessive sedation and hypoventilation. Heavy responsibility is placed on the ward nurses to both accurately assess the patient's level of pain and to deliver adequate analgesia. Repeatedly it has been shown that when pain relief is delegated to ward nurses, they fail to appreciate the degree of pain experienced by their patients, and administer inadequate doses of analgesics, often considerably less than prescribed.

Intermittent intravenous opioids prove little better than intramuscular opioids. Pain relief may be more rapid, but equally the rapidly achieved

peak serum concentration predisposes to somnolence. Continuous intravenous opioids tend to provide better relief of pain without marked fluctuations. Unfortunately when used alone progressive sedation is frequently
encountered.

In centres where equipment, monitoring facilities and staff shortages
prohibit the use of more invasive analgesic techniques, intermittent parenteral opioids can be successfully used in conjunction with simple methods of
local anaesthesia such as intercostal block.

The use of more sophisticated analgesia such as epidural and intrathecal
opioids is increasing in popularity. Often parenteral opioids are prescribed
for 'breakthrough' pain. Where such combinations are employed it is essential
that staff realize that the concomitant use of opioids by these routes significantly increases the risk of respiratory depression, especially in the elderly.

Epidural opioids

Epidural opioids have been used extensively since the discovery of spinal
opioid receptors. They have been shown to produce excellent analgesia
postoperatively following a wide range of procedures. Many opioids have
been investigated, though greatest experience exists with morphine.

It was hoped that epidural opioids would offer considerable advantages
over parenteral routes including: improved analgesia with smaller doses; a
localized effect; lack of motor and sympathetic block; and most important of
all, lack of respiratory depression. Unfortunately such optimism has not been
borne out by clinical experience. The greatest risk associated with epidural
opioids remains respiratory depression, which can occur many hours after
administration. Other less serious, though often distressing, side effects
include nausea, vomiting, pruritus, urinary retention and excessive sedation.
In an attempt to minimize these adverse effects various different opioids and
regimens have been investigated. The fact that so many different formula-
tions are currently used suggests that, for the present, no one opioid has an
outstanding advantage over another.

Mode of action

Opioids deposited in the epidural space, or directly into cerebrospinal
fluid (CSF) penetrate the spinal cord and exert their analgesic action by
binding with the pre-synaptic receptors in the substantia gelatinosa. Animal
experiments using radiolabelled C^{13} morphine demonstrated that the mor-

phine remained confined to the outer 1–2 mm of the spinal cord, even if sacrifice of the animal was delayed for several hours after morphine administration.

The extent to which epidural opioids exert their analgesic effect by systemic absorption is not clear. Some workers have found no difference in serum concentrations between epidurally and intravenously administered opioids for equianalgesia. Such findings have been confined to the highly lipophilic agents, such as fentanyl. With the hydrophilic agents most data would suggest a regional effect with considerably less opioid required by the epidural route than intravenous for comparable or improved pain relief. In fact serum levels below those known to produce analgesia are frequently reported with satisfactory pain relief.

Pharmacokinetics of epidural opioids

Opioids deposited in the epidural space must cross the dura, CSF and penetrate the spinal cord before binding to receptor sites. Factors which affect this transfer include the size and shape of the molecule, its lipid solubility and receptor affinity. Drugs of low molecular weight, elongated shape and which are highly lipophilic are the quickest to make this transfer with a clinical picture of rapid onset of analgesia. Drugs which remain in the epidural space for a long period of time due to low dural permeability characteristics may become bound to epidural fat, taken up by blood vessels or undergo metabolism. The clinical profile of these events is slow onset of analgesia and/or analgesia exerted by systemic effect.

Opioids which have penetrated the dura, or been directly deposited in the CSF, will bind with the spinal cord according to lipid solubility. Hydrophilic opioids such as morphine remain longer in the CSF and are subject to transportation to other sites by CSF circulation. The outcome is slow onset but prolonged and widespread analgesia, with the risk of rostral spread and possible respiratory depression.

The duration of action of opioids again relates to lipid solubility. Longest analgesic action is found with hydrophilic agents such as morphine and the shortest with lipophilic agents such as fentanyl. Diamorphine is an exception in that it has rapid onset of action due to its relatively high lipid solubility, but shows variable duration of action which may exceed morphine. This is probably due to its initial uptake into the spinal cord as diamorphine and continued action through hydrolysis to its active metabolites of mono-acetyl morphine and morphine.

Segmental effect

Epidural opioids have been shown to have a segmental effect. That is, an analgesic action confined closely to the area where the drug is deposited. First evidence of this effect was reported by Thompson *et al.* (1981) and Torda *et al.* (1980). The idea of segmental effect gave rise to the hypothesis that highly lipid-soluble opioids could be deposited in the thoracic region in the hope that analgesia would be maximum in this area, with minimum spread and reduced adverse effects.

It is difficult to draw realistic conclusions by comparing various published work on this subject, as there is obviously no standardization of method. Very few reports have been published using the same drug and dose, but at different levels of the epidural space, to evaluate segmental effect. Only two studies appear to have examined this issue, comparing fentanyl by lumbar and thoracic epidurals. Chamberlain *et al.* (1989) clearly demonstrated a segmental effect, but the sample size in each group was very small. Coe, *et al.* (1991) in a similar study using a much larger population, were unable to show any difference in pain scores, total dose of fentanyl required, or incidence of side effects. They concluded that no segmental effect was demonstrable. Whether segmental effect exists as a clinically relevant phenomenon is not yet established, although many workers continue to use highly lipophilic opioids via a thoracic epidural, confident in the advantages of segmental effect.

Choice of opioid

Most opioids have been given by the epidural route and effective analgesia reported. The main difficulty in comparing different opioids is in using equipotent doses. Equipotency between analgesics in the epidural space is not the same as for systemic use. Until data regarding this critical area are available it is difficult to draw useful clinical conclusions when comparing different agents.

The actual choice of opioid is therefore difficult. The decision is probably best determined by local conditions, that is, availability of equipment, nursing and medical personnel. Short-acting opioids require repeated boluses or continuous infusion. Longer-acting drugs can usually be given as a single bolus. Regardless of which agent is chosen, respiratory depression is always a possibility. It has been reported with all agents, and close observation is essential, probably for at least 12 hours after the last administered dose.

Site of access to epidural space

The epidural space can be approached in the cervical, thoracic, lumbar or caudal areas. Thoracic and lumbar approaches are the most commonly used for the relief of post-thoracotomy pain, although the caudal route has been successfully used.

Thoracic epidurals are widely used. The main questions pertaining to the thoracic epidural involve its safety, ease of cannulation and whether it holds significant advantages over lumbar epidural. Reports of neurological damage associated with thoracic epidurals are rare, although serious complications have occurred. The true incidence is likely to be less than reported in the medical literature due to medico-legal implications. Thoracic epidurals can be inserted with the patient awake or asleep. It is probably safer for the patient to be awake so that the cardinal sign of lancinating pain from cord puncture is not obscured by general anaesthesia.

Identification of the thoracic epidural space is more difficult than in the lumbar region due to steeper angulation of the spinous processes, and a paramedian approach is often necessary. In addition the epidural space is often shallower than in the lumbar region, making dural tap more likely. Failure to identify the space is reported at 2–10%, and must reflect anatomical difficulty, level of experience and a policy to accept failure early, rather than persevere and risk the consequences.

Whether there are any marked advantages of thoracic epidural over lumbar is debatable. Many practitioners would state that in capable hands the advantages far outweigh the small risk even with the patient asleep. Others are equally adamant in their view that blind invasion of the thoracic epidural space, especially in anaesthetized patients, can never be regarded as safe practice.

Intrathecal opioids

Intrathecal opioids, like epidural opioids, have been used to provide excellent pain relief following a wide range of surgical procedures. The mechanism of analgesia is probably the same for both, except for the variable systemic effect seen with epidural opioids.

As a technique the intrathecal route offers several advantages. Technically it is easier to perform with a definite end point. The total dose of opioid is considerably reduced, and dural permeability characteristics are eliminated. The potential for instrumental neurological damage is reduced and the onset of analgesia is rapid. It does however have several disadvantages. The length of effective analgesia is limited due to the one shot nature of the technique. This necessitates the use of long-acting opioids such as morphine, which is more susceptible to rostral spread and respiratory depression. If analgesia wears off leaving pain of such intensity as not to be controlled by simple analgesics, management becomes difficult. The subsequent use of parenteral opioids defeats the main point of using intrathecal analgesia and few anaesthetists are currently happy with the use of indwelling intrathecal catheters.

Individual patient opioid requirements vary immensely and the intrathecal route is a less forgiving technique than epidural. Inadvertent inappropriate dosage produces either short-term and/or inadequate analgesia, whilst overdose produces life-threatening respiratory depression. Gray *et al.* (1986) investigated the effect of baricity on duration of action. They found that hypobaric morphine had significantly longer analgesic effect than a hyperbaric solution, and that a mean dose of 0.79 mg had a mean duration of action of 22.9 hours. Unfortunately 84% of patients still required subsequent parenteral opioids.

Intrathecal opioids can provide excellent postoperative pain relief following thoracotomy, but the disadvantages of the technique seem to have limited its widespread use.

Complications of epidural and intrathecal opioids

Respiratory depression. All opioids, by whatever route, are capable of respiratory depression. The difference between agent and route is merely one of degree. Patients undergoing thoracic surgery frequently have pre-existing pulmonary disease, and the question of respiratory depression has special significance. Effective analgesia can limit postoperative hypoxaemia but respiratory depression is obviously counterproductive.

Criteria for definition of respiratory depression vary widely. Arterial carbon dioxide tension, respiratory rate, arterial saturation, peak expiratory flow rate, expiratory volume and forced vital capacity have all been used.

Whiting *et al.* (1988) have used respiratory inductive plethysmography to continuously monitor respiratory rate and periods of apnoea in patients post-thoracotomy. As a control for postoperative values a group of patients with COPD were studied during sleep, prior to surgery. 60% demonstrated episodes of apnoea (negligible tidal volume for > 15 seconds) and 20% had episodes of bradypnoea (respiratory rate < 10/min for > 5 minutes). This clearly emphasizes the abnormality of respiratory pattern which may be present in many patients undergoing thoracic surgery. Such factors need to be taken into account postoperatively when defining respiratory depression. In addition, postoperatively, they noted that three or more periods of apnoea per hour were associated with carbon dioxide retention and indicated significant respiratory depression. However, the number of episodes of bradypnoea was not a useful indicator of respiratory depression. As they rightly point out, discrete measurement of respiratory rate at specific time intervals will result in abnormalities of respiratory pattern being missed.

Respiratory depression has been reported with all opioids used by the epidural and intrathecal route, although in theory highly lipophilic agents should be associated with a lower risk. Factors which have been shown to predispose to respiratory depression include advanced age, use of hydrophilic opioids, concomitant use of parenteral opioids, intrathecal and thoracic epidural administration.

Attempts to reduce the incidence of respiratory depression have included infusions of naloxone and opioid agonist/antagonists such as nalbuphine. Both have been reported as successful but analgesia may be reduced, therefore complicating management.

Because of the potential for respiratory depression, patients who have received epidural or intrathecal opioids should be nursed in areas with adequate nursing staff, monitoring equipment and rapid access to medical assistance. Continuous monitoring of arterial saturation, end tidal carbon dioxide and respiratory rate is attractive, but it is the interpretation and trend of data which are as critical as the absolute values. Whatever equipment is used, it is the continuous presence of experienced staff who appreciate the potential problems that is by far the most important.

Urinary retention. Urinary retention following any surgery is not uncommon. Its occurrence is, however, markedly increased by the use of epidural or intrathecal opioids and local anaesthetic blocks. Reported incidences range from 6–72%. Some centres have found it sufficiently troublesome as to routinely catheterize all patients receiving epidural analgesia.

Local anaesthetic block of sacral segments (S_{2-4}) results in bladder atonia. Block of T_{12} and L_1 increases bladder sphincter tone by abolishing reflex activity. Retention precipitated by local anaesthetics alone is often painless, and does not respond to opioid antagonists. Other than waiting for the effect of the local anaesthetic to wear off, recourse to catheterization is the only option.

Epidural opioids cause marked relaxation of the detrusor muscle leading to increased maximum bladder capacity and retention. The effect may result from interference with sacral parasympathetic outflow. Young men appear particularly susceptible and an incidence of 90% has been reported in this group. Naloxone in small titrated doses may relieve retention associated with opioids, but it is not always successful and can reverse analgesia.

Pruritus. Pruritus can occur after administration of opioids by any route, but it is much more common after epidural or intrathecal administration. The reported incidences vary from 5–70%. The itching usually begins within 1–3 hours, and is not confined to any segmental area of action of the opioid. The intensity varies considerably, many patients only admitting to it on direct questioning, which must be a factor affecting the discrepancy of reported incidence. It is unclear if the pruritus is an age-, drug-, dose- or gender-related phenomenon. It has been suggested that parturients are particularly susceptible.

The mechanism is not known. It is postulated that the phenomenon is due to histamine release and proportional to the concentration of drug at the mast cell membrane. Others have suggested that itching results from the effect of the opioid on the trigeminal nucleus causing sensory modulation. No consistent elevation of serum histamine is found in patients complaining of pruritus, although this does not rule out the role of local tissue histamine release. It is interesting to note that a large proportion of patients obtain relief of symptoms with antihistamines whilst complete resolution can be achieved with naloxone.

Both infusions of naloxone and nalbuphine have been reported to reduce the severity and incidence of pruritus, but as with similar efforts to reduce respiratory depression, it complicates treatment, is not always successful and may reduce analgesia.

Patient-controlled analgesia

One of the major advances in the relief of postoperative pain to emerge in the last decade has been the introduction of patient-controlled analgesia (PCA). Various different commercial apparatus exists but the basic principle allows patients to demand analgesia from the equipment, as necessary to relieve their pain, up to a pre-set limit of both dose and time. The hope, which has been predominantly borne out, is that patients will optimize their analgesia while minimizing adverse effects. Several opioids have been used but most experience exists with morphine and fentanyl.

There is mounting experience with PCA, and almost without exception, excellent results are reported both in terms of analgesia and patient acceptance. The main advantage lies in the flexibility of the technique with regard to differences in pharmacokinetics and pharmacodynamics of opioids between individuals. Success of PCA also seems to be in the attitude of patients. Anxiety is reduced as patients feel in control of their pain, and have peace of mind in the knowledge that analgesics are 'freely' available. Inhibited patients feel less of a nuisance and potential embarrassment about analgesic requirements is eliminated. PCA however is not suitable for all patients. The frail, very elderly and confused in particular do not make appropriate use of PCA.

Experience with PCA in the management of post-thoracotomy patients is not extensive, but results are encouraging. Lange *et al.* (1988) demonstrated fewer X-ray changes postoperatively in patients using PCA, compared to a control group, and Keeri-Szanto (1984) has reported a reduced hospital stay of 22% after thoracotomy in patients using PCA, compared with conventional treatment.

PCA devices which register requests for analgesia which are denied, due to the pre-set lockout time or total dosage, provide information regarding level of analgesia. In addition they provide a new method of assessing different techniques of pain relief. The amount of analgesia requested and supplied by the PCA device, whilst receiving the method of pain relief under investigation, provides objective information about the efficacy of analgesia under evaluation.

PCA has also been used to control epidural opioid infusions. Fentanyl appears to be the most popular choice, and probably the most suitable given its rapid onset of action. Published work is still limited, but Grant *et al.* (1990) reported improved analgesia, lower carbon dioxide tension and reduced total fentanyl requirements following thoracotomy, when compared to intravenous PCA fentanyl.

PCA is not automatic analgesia. It requires the presence of informed and dedicated staff both medical and nursing. Patients require instruction pre- and postoperatively. Staff need to supervise the patient and adjust programming of the device in the light of clinical circumstances. Complications of opioid administration will still arise, although it is hoped less frequently, but sustained vigilance by all staff is still required.

Transdermal opioids

Transdermal administration of opioids is a new area in analgesia. Fentanyl has been formulated in a transdermal preparation which, when applied to a hair-free patch of skin on the chest, delivers fentanyl at an approximate rate of 100 µg/hour. Its role in postoperative pain management is not yet fully evaluated. It is an attractive concept in its simplicity, but may be subject to variable absorption and cannot be titrated.

Serum levels are slow to reach steady-state and the patch would need to be applied several hours preoperatively. An intravenous bolus of fentanyl at induction will also be required if analgesic levels are to be achieved by the end of surgery. When Gourlay *et al.* (1989) applied the patch at the time of induction, despite a loading intravenous dose of 100–200 µg, a mean delay of 12.7 hours elapsed before minimum effective blood concentration (MEC) was reached!

Another factor which may limit its use, especially in thoracic surgery, is the continued absorption after removal of the patch, from the deposit of fentanyl formed in the skin. Gourlay *et al.* (1989) also examined this problem and found a mean delay of 16 hours before blood concentrations fell below MEC, after removal of the patch. Management of excessive sedation or respiratory depression becomes difficult in this situation, and recourse to the use of naloxone more likely.

OTHER FORMS OF ANALGESIA

Cryoanalgesia

Cold has been used for centuries for its ability to reduce pain. In 1976 Lloyd *et al.* described the specific application of extreme cold to nerves to achieve analgesia by means of a long-term but ultimately reversible nerve block, naming the technique cryoanalgesia. They included its application to intercostal nerves during thoracotomy and so established the procedure which gained considerable popularity during the 1980s and is still widely used.

The cryoprobe is based on the Joule–Thompson principle in which, when high pressure gas is allowed to expand within the probe tip, rapid cooling to freezing temperatures occurs. The most commonly used gas is nitrous oxide which permits temperatures of $-20°C$ to $-60°C$ to be achieved. The probe is applied directly to the nerve as close as possible to the intercostal foramen, and proximal to the collateral branches. Freezing for 30–60 seconds is permitted. The ice-ball which forms must be allowed to thaw before removal of the probe, to prevent avulsion of the nerve. A second application is sometimes used. The nerve at the level of the incision (usually T_5), plus at least two adjacent nerves above and below, receive such treatment, but up to eight intercostal nerves can be treated. It is important that the anaesthetized area includes the sites for chest drain insertion.

Cryoanalgesia achieved popularity as a technique because it was easy to perform, adds only minutes to the operating time, does not require intensive observation postoperatively and is without serious side effects, namely respiratory depression and sympathetic blockade. As a form of pain relief one can predict it will be inadequate as the sole means of analgesia. Cryoanalgesia does not affect the posterior primary rami of the intercostal nerves supplying the posterior aspect of the chest. In addition, apical chest drains may irritate unfrozen segments of the pleura, and it will have no effect on pain arising from the shoulder joint or noxious stimuli conducted via the phrenic and vagus nerve. It would be reasonable to assume that cryoanalgesia can at best only act as an adjunct to some other form of pain relief.

Studies using cryoanalgesia give conflicting results. Early reports were promising, showing improved pain relief and decreased supplementary analgesic requirements. Unfortunately these frequently quoted studies failed to include control groups, or omitted data regarding means of assessing pain relief. Roberts *et al.* (1988) did, however, show an advantage of cryoanalgesia over intercostal nerve blocks with local anaesthesia and Orr *et al.* (1981) found improved pain relief when compared to intramuscular morphine as the sole analgesic. Others, including Roxburgh *et al.* (1987) failed to find any beneficial effect of cryoanalgesia when used to supplement extradural opioids. Muller *et al.* (1989) likewise failed to detect any significant difference between pain, additional analgesic requirements and forced expiratory flow rate, compared to control groups. It is possible that earlier studies of cryoanalgesia found a beneficial effect compared to the standard analgesic options available, those being predominantly intramuscular opioids and single shot intercostal nerve blocks. With advances and increasing confidence in analgesic techniques, such as epidural opioids and extrapleural catheters, the role of cryoanalgesia is diminishing.

The advantages of cryoanalgesia have probably been overstated, and the assumption of being without serious side effects unfounded. Paresis of both intercostal and abdominal muscles in the early postoperative period may impair peak expiratory flow and reduce effective coughing. The length of time to regeneration of the nerve and normal sensation is unpredictable, and nerve damage may be permanent. Anaesthesia of the breast and nipple is often distressing, especially in young women, and poses specific reflex problems with subsequent breastfeeding. But perhaps the most worrying aspect is the long-term consequences of cryoanalgesia and the development of neuralgia (see chronic post-thoracotomy pain, p. 122). One must conclude that the place of cryoanalgesia is questionable. There is little evidence of any advantage when combined with more invasive analgesic techniques and it is inadequate when used alone.

Non-steroidal anti-inflammatory drugs

Non-steroidal anti-inflammatory drugs (NSAIDs) are used to treat mild to moderate pain. Alone they have insufficient analgesic action to control pain following major surgery. Several reports have shown an opioid sparing effect when used for postoperative relief of pain. These effects have also been reported in the management of post-thoracic surgical pain. All reports have shown significantly reduced requirements for opioid analgesia, lower pain scores and reduced pain on movement and coughing compared to control groups. In addition no adverse effects were reported with the short-term use of NSAIDs, although all excluded patients with a history of peptic ulceration.

NSAIDs interfere with normal platelet function, and may result in increased blood loss intraoperatively. In addition, NSAIDs have recently been associated with the onset of renal failure. For this reason they are probably best avoided in those with pre-existing renal dysfunction and limited to the first few days after surgery.

The choice of NSAID is probably unimportant given the reported success of several agents. Diclofenac has the advantage of being long acting and available in oral, intramuscular and suppository form. NSAIDs are not without side effects, but appear a very useful adjunct to other forms of analgesia.

Nitrous oxide

Nitrous oxide is frequently used intraoperatively, and whilst only a weak analgesic, it may provide some useful analgesia in the very early postoperative period. Patient-controlled mixtures of nitrous oxide and oxygen (Entonox) are useful in the postoperative period, providing short periods of additional analgesia during removal of chest drains and during physiotherapy.

Clonidine

Clonidine is an α-adrenoceptor agonist with proven analgesic action. Its analgesic effect is reversed by β-blocking drugs but not naloxone. Clonidine has been shown to produce analgesia in postoperative patients when given intravenously and epidurally. In addition clonidine and morphine appear to have a synergistic effect.

Its use in the management of post-thoracotomy pain is not established. Gordh (1988) failed to find any additional analgesic action with 3 μg/kg of epidurally administered clonidine compared to a control group. However, a significant depression in systolic blood pressure was noted, though no patient required treatment for hypotension. No other side effects were noted. As Gordh points out, the analgesic action of clonidine may be insufficient to treat the intense pain associated with thoracotomy. No other reports of the use of clonidine for post-thoracic surgical pain relief have appeared in the literature, but further investigations of this interesting agent, especially its synergistic action with morphine, are warranted.

Transcutaneous nerve stimulation

Transcutaneous nerve stimulation (TENS) is a non-invasive method of pain relief, based on the gate theory of pain. There are no apparent serious side effects associated with its use. The only absolute contraindication is the presence of a permanent pacemaker. Several reports using TENS have shown a reduction in opioid requirement following a variety of surgical procedures including orthopaedic, obstetric, gynaecological and abdominal surgery. In addition some other workers have reported improved respiratory function and decreased incidence of nausea and vomiting. Others have failed to confirm these findings.

Several investigations of TENS in post-thoracic pain have reported on opioid requirements. Warfield *et al.* (1985) found no difference in opioid requirement but significantly lower pain scores. Rooney *et al.* (1983) found that five patients in a TENS group of 22 required no opioid analgesia on the first postoperative day, compared to all the control group who did require opioid supplements. More recently Stubbings and Jellicoe (1988) failed to find any difference between TENS and a control group with regard to opioid requirements, quality of pain relief, site of pain or peak expiratory flow rate. In fact the only advantage they could elucidate was a reduced incidence of nausea and vomiting in the study group.

The advantages of TENS, if any, are difficult to prove, but given its innocuous nature it certainly does no harm, and may in certain individuals prove highly effective.

Acupuncture

Acupuncture is a traditional Chinese therapy best known in Western medicine for its analgesic properties. It has been used in a wide variety of surgical conditions including thoracotomy. Proposed mechanisms of action include placebo effect, stimulation of endogenous opioids and activation of the gate control mechanism. In China it has been used as the sole anaesthetic for thoracotomy with the patient remaining conscious throughout surgery!

Its use in Western medicine in acute pain control is unfortunately limited by lack of experienced practitioners.

CONCLUSION

The pain which occurs following thoracotomy can be managed by a vast number of techniques either alone or in combinations. The appearance of relatively new methods such as intrapleural, extrapleural and patient-controlled analgesia should prompt many anaesthetists involved in the management of such patients to critically evaluate the level of analgesia afforded to their patients. There is still no outstanding analgesic regimen hence the range of options and volumes of literature generated on the subject.

In attempting to formulate the optimum analgesic practice by rational consideration of the different published work several difficulties arise. These include:

non-standardization of anaesthetic technique;

differing methods of pain assessment (e.g. visual analogue scale vs verbal ranking score);

effect of local anaesthesia established prior to surgical stimuli;

differing criteria for definition of respiratory depression;

method of eliciting side effects (i.e. direct questioning vs spontaneously offered information);

incidence of urinary retention difficult to evaluate with some units routinely catheterizing all thoracic surgery patients.

Despite the vast array of analgesic techniques now available to anaesthetists in this area, a consensus of opinion is beginning to emerge. The concept of 'balanced' analgesia is gaining popularity. That is, a multidirectional approach towards pain, rather than relying on a single mode of analgesia. The desired result is to reduce pain and concomitant side effects. A combination of an opioid, local anaesthesia and NSAIDs possibly holds the most promise at present. The ideal form of administering the local anaesthetic and opioid is not decided. Epidural, extrapleural and paravertebral approaches are all promising. Whether or not analgesia should be commenced before the onset of surgical stimuli is not known, but animal experimentation and clinical impression would suggest that this is the case.

Consideration of immediate postoperative pain is the main emphasis of current clinical work-though increasing interest is being directed towards the occurrence of long-term pain not related to the original pathology. The outcome of work relating to long-term pain may well alter the manner in which we treat patients postoperatively. For the present we must await the long-term follow-up of the various innovative forms of pain relief.

FURTHER READING

Postoperative management

Craig D.B. (1981) Post operative recovery of pulmonary function. *Anesthesia and Analgesia*, **60**, 46–52.

Goldstraw P.G. (1987) Post-operative management of the thoracic surgical patient. In: Gothard J.W.W. (ed.) *Thoracic Anaesthesia. Clinical Anaesthesiology*, Vol. 1, pp. 207–231. Baillière Tindall, London.

Hallfeldt K.K.J., Knoefel W.T., Thetter O. & Schweiber L. (1990) *Heart and Lung*, **19**, 432 [letter].

Pandid S.K., Galway J.E. & Dundee J.W. (1973) Acidosis following thoracic surgery. *British Journal of Anaesthesia*, **45**, 79–85.

Dysrhythmias

Borgeat A., Biollaz J., Bayer-Berger M., Kappenberger L., Chapius G. & Chiolér R. (1989) Prevention of dysrhythmias by flecainide after non-cardiac thoracic surgery. *Annals of Thoracic Surgery*, **48**, 232–234.

Borgeat A., Petropoutos P., Cavin R., Biollaz J., Munofa A. & Schwander D. (1991) Prevention of dysrhythmias after non cardiac thoracic operations. Flecainide versus digoxin. *Annals of Thoracic Surgery*, **51**, 964–968.

Echt D.S., Liebson P.R., Mitchell L.B. *et al.* (1991) Mortality and morbidity in patients receiving encainide, flecainide or placebo. The cardiac arrhythmia suppression trial. *New England Journal of Medicine*, **34**, 781–788.

Ghosh P. & Pakrashi B.C. (1972) Cardiac dysrhythmias after thoracotomy. *British Heart Journal*, **34**, 374–376.

Krowka M.J., Paivolero P.C., Trastek R.F., Payne W.S. & Bernatz P.E. (1987) Cardiac dysrhythmias following pneumonectomy. Clinical correlates and prognostic significance. *Chest*, **91**, 490–495.

Momory F. & Reynolds E.F. (1964) Cardiac rhythm disturbances complicating resectional surgery of the lung. *Annals of Internal Medicine*, **61**, 688–695.

Ritchie A.J., Bowe P. & Gibbons J.R.P. (1990) Prophylactic digitalization for thoracotomy: a reassessment. *Annals of Thoracic Surgery*, **50**, 86–88.

Alteration in respiratory mechanics following thoracic surgery

Bartlett R.H., Brennan M.C., Gassaniga A.B. & Hanson E.L. (1973) Studies on the pathogenesis and prevention of post-operative pulmonary complications. *Surgery, Gynecology and Obstetrics*, **137**, 925–933.

Bartlett, R.M. (1980) Pulmonary pathophysiology in surgical patients. *Surgical Clinics of North America*, **60**, 1323–1338.

Craig D.B. (1981) Post operative recovery of pulmonary function. See under Postoperative Management.

Entwistle M.D., Roe P.G., Sapsford D.J., Berisford R.G. & Jones J.G. (1991) Patterns of oxygenation after thoracotomy. *British Journal of Anaesthesia*, **67**, 704–711.

Leblanc P., Ruff F. & Milic-Emil J. (1970) Effects of age and body position on airway closure in man. *Journal of Applied Physiology*, **28**, 448–451.

Lutchen K.R., Saidel G.M., Prmiano F.P., Horowitz S.G. & Deal E.C. (1984) Mechanics and gas distribution in normal and obstructed lungs during tidal breathing. *American Review of Respiratory Disease*, **130**, 974–979.

Rehder Der K., Cameron P.D. & Krayer S. (1985) New dimensions of the respiratory system. *Anesthesiology*, **62**, 230–233.

Sabanathan S., Eng J. & Mearns A.J. (1990) Alteration in respiratory mechanics following thoracotomy. *Journal of the Royal College of Surgeons of Edinburgh*, **35**, 144–150.

Physiotherapy

Craig D.B. (1981) Post operative recovery of pulmonary function. See under Postoperative Management.

Craven J.L., Evans G.A., Davenport P.J. & Williams R.H.P. (1974) The evaluation of incentive spirometry in the management of post-operative pulmonary complications. *British Journal of Surgery*, **61**, 793–797.

Frolund L. & Madsen F. (1986) Self administered prophylactic post-operative positive expiratory pressure in thoracic surgery. *Acta Anaesthesiologica Scandinavica*, **30**, 381–385.

Paul W.L. & Downs J.B. (1981) Post-operative atelectasis: intermittent pressure breathing, incentive spirometry and face-mask positive end-expiratory pressure. *Archives of Surgery*, **116**, 861–863.

Pinilla J.C., Olenik F.H., Tan L. *et al.* (1990) Use of a nasal continuous positive airway pressure mask in the treatment of post-operative atelectasis in aortocoronary bypass surgery. *Critical Care Medicine*, **18**, 836–840.

Postoperative analgesia

The Royal College of Surgeons of England and the College of Anaesthetists (1990) *Commission on the Provision of Surgical Services: Report of the Working Party on Pain After Surgery*, London

Donovan M., Dillon P. & McGuire L. (1987) Incidence and characteristics of pain in a sample of medico-surgical in-patients. *Pain*, **30**, 69–78.

Grant B.P., Dolman J.F., Harper J.A. *et al.* (1990) Patient controlled lumbar epidural fentanyl for post-thoracotomy pain. *Canadian Journal of Anaesthesia*, **37**, 945.

Keeri-Szanto M. (1990) New analgesic agents and techniques shorten post-operative hospital stay. *Pain*, **2**, S 397.

Loan W.B. & Morrison J.B. (1967) The incidence and severity of post-operative pain. *British Journal of Anaesthesia*, **39**, 695–698.

Ready, L.B. (1990) Patient controlled analgesia — does it provide more than comfort? *Canadian Journal of Anaesthesia*, **37**, 719–721.

New concepts in pain.

Conacher I.D. (1986) Percutaneous cryotherapy for post-thoracotomy neuralgia. *Pain*, **25**, 227–228.

McQuay H.J. & Dickenson A.H. (1990) Implications of nervous system plasticity for pain management. *Anaesthesia*, **45**, 101–102.

Woolf C.J. (1989) Recent advances in the pathophysiology of acute pain. *British Journal of Anaesthesia*, **63**, 139–146.

Chronic post-thoracotomy pain

Conacher I.D. (1986) Percutaneous cryotherapy for post-thoracotomy neuralgia. *Pain*, **2**, 227–228.

Conacher I.D., Locke T. & Milton C. (1986) Neuralgia after cryoanalgesia for thoracotomy. *Lancet*, **1**, 277.

Dajczman E., Gordon A., Kreisman H. & Wolkore N. (1991) Long term post-thoracotomy pain. *Chest*, **99**, 270–274.

Johannesen N., Madsen G. & Ahlburg P. (1990) Neurological sequelae after cryoanalgesia for thoracotomy pain relief. *Annales Chirurgiae et Gynaecologiae*, **79**, 108–109.

Kalso E., Perttinen K. & Kadsinen S. (1992) Pain after thoracic surgery. *Acta Anaesthesiologica Scandinavica*, **36**, 96–100.

Matsunaga M., Dan K. & Hara F. (1990) Residual pain of 90 thoracotomy patients with malignancy and non-malignancy. *Pain*, **5**, 149.

Muller L. Ch., Salzer G.M., Ramaur G. & Neiss A. (1989) Intraoperative cryoanalgesia for post-thoracotomy pain relief. *Annals of Thoracic Surgery*, **48**, 8–15.

Roxburgh D., Markland C.G., Ross B.A. & Kerr W.F. (1987) Role of cryoanalgesia in the control of pain after thoracotomy. *Thorax*, **42**, 292–295.

Intercostal nerve block

Kolvenbach H., Lauven P.M., Schneider B. & Kunath U. (1989) Repetitive intercostal nerve block via catheter for post-operative pain relief after thoracotomy. *Thoracic Cardiovascular Surgery*, **37**, 273–276.

Safran D., Kuhlman G., Orhant E.E., Castelain M.H. & Journois D. (1990) Continuous intercostal blockade with lidocaine after thoracic surgery. *Anesthesia and Analgesia*, **70**, 345–349.

Extrapleural analgesia

Mozell E.J., Sabanathan S., Mearns A.J., Bickford-Smith P.J., Majid M.R. & Zografos G. (1991) Continuous extrapleural intercostal nerve block after pleurectomy. *Thorax*, **46**, 21–24.

Sabanathan S., Mearns A.J., Bickford-Smith P.J. *et al.* (1990) Efficacy of continuous extrapleural intercostal nerve block on post-thoracotomy pain and pulmonary mechanics. *British Journal of Surgery*, **77**, 221–225.

Intrapleural analgesia

Ferrante F.M., Vincent N.S., Arthur G.R. & Rocco A.G. (1991) Intrapleural analgesia after thoracotomy. *Anesthesia and Analgesia*, **72**, 105–109.

Kambam J.R., Hammon J., Parris W.V.C. & Lupinetti F.M. (1989) Intrapleural analgesia for post-thoracotomy pain and blood levels of bupivacaine following intrapleural injection. *Canadian Journal of Anaesthesia*, **36**, 106–109.

Rosenberg P.H., Scheinin B.M.A., Lepantalo M.J.A. & Lindfors O. (1987) Continuous intrapleural infusion of bupivacaine for analgesia after thoracotomy. *Anesthesiology*, **67**, 811–813.

Symreng T., Gomez M.N., Johnson B. & Rossi N.P. (1988) Intrapleural bupivacaine vs. saline after thoracotomy — effects on pain and lung function — a double blind study. *Anesthesia and Analgesia*, **67**, S1–S266.

Paravertebral block

Conacher I.D. & Kokri M. (1987) Post-operative para-vertebral blocks for thoracic surgery. *British Journal of Anaesthesia*, **59**, 155–161.

Matthews P.J. & Govenden V. (1989) Comparison of continuous paravertebral and extradural infusions of bupivacaine for pain relief after thoracotomy. *British Journal of Anaesthesia*, **62**, 204–205.

Purcell-Jones G., Pither C.E. & Justins D.M. (1987) Para-vertebral block — a misnomer? (In: Abstracts from scientific papers.) *6th Annual Meeting of the European Society of Regional Anaesthesia*, 182.

Epidural local anaesthetics

Bokesch P.M., Raymond S.A. & Strichartz G. (1987) Dependency of lidocaine potency on pH and PCO_2. *Anesthesia and Analgesia*, **66**, 9–17.

George K.A., Wright P.M.C. & Chisakuta A. (1991) Continuous thoracic epidural fentanyl for post-thoracotomy pain relief, with or without bupivacaine. *Anesthesiology*, **46**, 732–736.

Logas W.G., El-Baz N. & El-Garizonio A. *et al.* (1987) Continuous thoracic epidural analgesia for post-operative pain relief following thoracotomy: a randomised prospective study. *Anesthesiology*, **67**, 787–791.

McMorland G.M., Douglas M.J., Ross P.E.E. *et al.* (1986) Effect of pH adjustment of bupivacaine on onset and duration of epidural analgesia in parturients. *Canadian Anaesthetists Society Journal*, **33**, **5**, 537–41.

Wattwill M., Sundberg A., Arvill A. & Lennquist C. (1985) Circulatory changes during high thoracic epidural anaesthesia. Influence of sympathetic block and of systemic effect of the local anaesthetic. *Acta Anaesthesiologica, Scandinavica*, **29**, 849–855.

Epidural opioids

Bonica J.J., Backup P.H., Anderson C.E., Hadfield D., Crepps W.F. & Mowc B.F. (1957) Peridural block: analysis of 3,637 cases and review. *Anesthesiology*, **18**, 723–784.

Brodsky J.B., Kretzschmar K.M. & Mark J.B.D. (1988) Caudal epidural morphine for post-thoracotomy pain. *Anesthesia and Analgesia*, **67**, 409–410.

Bromage P.R. (1989) The control of post-thoracotomy pain. *Anaesthesia*, **44**, 445–446.

Chamberlain D.P., Bodily M.N., Olssen G.L. & Ramsey D.M. (1989) Comparison of lumbar vs. thoracic epidural fentanyl for post-thoracotomy analgesia using patient controlled dosage. *Regional Anaesthesia*, (Suppl.) **14**, 26.

Coe A., Sarginson R., Smith M.W., Donnelly R.J. & Russell G.N. (1991) Pain following thoracotomy. *Anaesthesia*, **46**, 918–921.

Grant B.P., Dolman J.F., Harper J.A. *et al.* (1990) Patient controlled lumbar epidural fentanyl for post-thoracotomy pain. *Canadian Journal of Anaesthesia*, **37**, 345.

Morgan M. (1989) The rational use of intrathecal and extradural opioids. *British Journal of Anaesthesia*, **63**, 165–188.

Nordberg G., Hedner T., Melltrand T. & Dahlstrom B. (1983) Pharmacokinetic aspects of epidural morphine analgesia. *Anesthesiology*, **58**, 545–551.

Panos L., Sadler A.N., Stringer D.G., Badner N., Lawson S. & Koren G. (1990) Continuous infusions of lumbar epidural fentanyl and intravenous fentanyl for post-thoracotomy pain relief. Analgesia and pharmacokinetic effects. *Canadian Journal of Anaesthesia*, **37**, 566.

Thompson W.R., Smith P.T., Hirst M., Varkey G.P. & Icnill R.C. (1981) Regional analgesic effect of epidural morphine in volunteers. *Canadian Anaesthetists Society Journal*, **28**, 530–536.

Torda T.A., Pybus D.A., Lieberman H., Clark M. & Crawford M. (1980) Experimental comparison of extradural and intramuscular morphine. *British Journal of Anaesthesia*, **52**, 939–943.

Vaughan R.S. & Gough J.D. (1989) The control of post-thoracotomy pain. *Anaesthesia*, **44**, 445–446.

Weddel S.J. & Ritter R.R. (1981) Serum levels following epidural administration of morphine and correlation with pain relief of post-surgical pain. *Anesthesiology*, **54**, 210–214.

Yaksh T.L. (1983) The principles behind the use of spinal narcotics. *Clinics in Anaesthesiology*, **1**, 219–232.

Intrathecal opioids

Gray J.R., Fromme G.A., Nauss L.A., Wang J.K. & Ilstop D.M. (1986) Intrathecal morphine for post-thoracotomy pain. *Anesthesia and Analgesia*, **65**, 873–876.

Complications of epidural and intrathecal opioids

Baxter A.D., Samson B. & Doren R. (1989) Prevention of epidural morphine induced respiratory depression with intravenous nalbuphine infusion in post-thoracotomy patients. *Canadian Journal of Anaesthesia*, **36**, 503–509.

Bromage P.R. (1981) The price of intraspinal narcotics: basic constraints. *Anesthesia and Analgesia*, **60**, 461–463.

Bromage P.R., Camporesi E.M., Durant P.A.C. & Nielson C.H. (1982) Non respiratory side effects of epidural morphine. *Anesthesia and Analgesia*, **61**, 490–495.

Hobbs G.J. & Roberts F.L. (1992) Epidural infusion of bupivacaine and diamorphine for post-operative analgesia. *Anaesthesia*, **47**, 58–62.

Korsh (1987) Systemic histamine release by epidural morphine. *Anesthesiology*, **67**, A475.

Morgan M. (1989) The rational use of intrathecal and extradural opioids. See under Epidural Opioids.

Penning J.P., Samson B. & Baxter A.D. (1988) Reversal of epidural morphine induced respiratory depression and pruritus with nalbuphine. *Canadian Journal of Anaesthesia*, **35**, 599–605.

Rawal N., Mollefors K., Axelsson K., Ligardh G. & Widman B. (1983) An experimental study of urodynamic effects of epidural morphine and naloxone reversal. *Anesthesia and Analgesia*, **62**, 641–647.

Rawal N., Schott V., Danlstrom B. *et al.* (1986) Influence of naloxone infusion on analgesia and respiratory depression following epidural morphine. *Anesthesiology*, **64**, 194–201.

Roscow C.E., Moss J. & Philbin D.M. (1982) Histamine release during morphine and fentanyl anaesthesia. *Anesthesiology*, **56**, 93–96.

Shipton E.A. (1984) Pruritus — a side effect of epidural fentanyl for post-operative analgesia. *South African Medical Journal*, **66**, 61–2.

Whiting W.C., Sandler A.N., Lan L.C., Chovaz P.M., Slavchenko P., Daley D. & Koren G. (1988) Analgesia and respiratory effects of epidural sufentanil in patients following thoracotomy. *Anesthesiology*, **69**, 36–43.

Patient-controlled analgesia

Grant R.P. *et al.* (1990) Patient controlled lumbar epidural fentanyl for post-thoracotomy pain. See under Epidural Opioids.

Keeri-Szanto M. (1984) New analgesic agents and techniques shorten post-operative hospital stay. *Pain*, **2**, S 397.

Lange M.P., Dahn M.S. & Jacobs L.A. (1988) Patient controlled analgesia vs. intermittent analgesia dosing. *Heart and Lung*, **17**, 495–498.

Ready L.B. (1990) Patient controlled analgesia — does it provide more than comfort? *Canadian Journal of Anaesthesia*, **37**, 719–721.

Transdermal Opioids

Duthie D.J.R., Rowbothan D.J., Wyld R., Henderson P.D. & Nimmo W.S. (1988) Plasma fentanyl concentrations during transdermal delivery of fentanyl to surgical patients. *British Journal of Anaesthesia*, **60**, 614–618.

Gourlay G.K., Kowalski S.R., Plummer J.L., Cherry D.A., Gaukroger P. & Cousins M.J. (1989) The transdermal administration of fentanyl in the treatment of post-operative pain; pharmacokinetic and pharmacodynamic effects. *Pain*, **37**, 193–202.

Cryoanalgesia

Conacher I.D. (1990) Pain relief after thoracotomy. *British Journal of Anaesthesia*, **65**, 806–812.
Lloyd J.W.., Barnard J.D.W. & Glynn C.J. (1976) Cryoanalgesia, a new approach to analgesia. *The Lancet*. **30**, 932–934.
Maiwand M.O. & Makey A.R. (1981) Cryoanalgesia for pain relief after thoracotomy. *British Medical Journal*, **282** 1749–1750.
Maiwand M.O., Makey A.R. & Rees A. (1986) Cryoanalgesia after thoracotomy. *Journal of Thoracic and Cardiovascular Surgery*, **92**, 291–296.
Orr I.A., Keenan D.J.M. & Dundee J.W. (1981) Improved pain relief after thoracotomy. Use of cryoprobe and morphine infusion. *British Medical Journal*, **283**, 945.
Roberts D., Pizzarelli Lepore V., Alkhaja N., Belboul A. & Darnevik L. (1988) Reduction of post thoracotomy pain by cryotherapy of intercostal nerves. *Scandinavian Journal of Thoracic and Cardiovascular Surgery*, **22**, 127–130.
Also see references under Chronic Post-Thoracotomy Pain.

Non-steroidal anti-inflammatory drugs

Gilles G.W., Kenny G.N., Bullingham R.E. & McArdale C.S. (1987) The morphine sparing effect of ketorolac trimethamine. A study of a new parenteral non-steroidal anti-inflammatory agent after abdominal surgery. *Anaesthesia*, **42**, 727–731.
Jones R.M., Cashman J.N., Foster J.M., Nedley J.R. & Adams A.P. (1985) Comparison of infusions of morphine and lysine acetyl salicylate for relief of pain following thoracic surgery. *British Journal of Anaesthesia*, **57**, 259–263.
Keenan D.J.M., Cave K., Langdon L. & Lea R.E. (1983) Comparative trial of rectal indomethacin and cryoanalgesia for control of early post-thoracotomy pain. *British Medical Journal*, **287**, 1335–1337.
McQuay H.J. & Dickenson A.H. (1990). Implications of nervous system plasticity for pain management. See under New Concepts in Pain.
Owen H., Glavin R.J. & Shaw N.A. (1986) Ibuprofen in the management of post-operative pain. *British Journal of Anaesthesia*, **58**, 1371–1375.
Pavy T., Medley C. & Murphy D.F. (1990) Effects of indomethacin on pain relief after thoracotomy. *British Journal of Anaesthesia*, **65**, 624–627.

Clonidine

Carabine V.A., Milligan K.R. & Moore J. (1992) Extradural clonidine and bupivacaine for post-operative analgesia. *British Journal of Anaesthesia*, **68**, 132–136.
Gordh Jr. T. (1988) Epidural clonidine for treatment of post-operative pain after thoraco-tomy. *Acta Anaesthesiologica Scandinavica*, **32**, 702–709.
Gordh Jr. T. & Tamsen A. (1983) A study of the analgesic effect of clonidine in man. *Acta Anaesthesiologica Scandinavica*, **27**, 72.
Kalia P.K., Madan R., Batgra R.K., Latha V., Vardman W. & Gode G.R. (1986) Clinical study on epidural clonidine for post-operative analgesia. *Indian Journal of Medical Research*, **83**, 550–552.

Nalda M.A. & Gonzalez J.L. (1986) Post-operative pain relief with synergistic interaction of epidural clonidine and morphine (abstr.). In: Bergman H. & Icramar H. (eds) *7th European Congress of Anaesthesiology*, **11**, 262.

Transcutaneous nerve stimulation

Neary J.M. (1981) TENS for relief of post-incisional surgical pain. *American Association of Nurses and Anesthetists Journal*, **49**, 151–155.

Rooney S.M., Jain S. & Goldiner P.L. (1983) Effects of TENS on post-operative pain after thoracotomy. *Anesthesia and Analgesia*, **62**, 1010–1012.

Stubbings J.F. & Jellicoe J.A. (1988) TENS after thoracotomy. *Anaesthesia*, **43**, 296–298.

Van Derark G.D. & McGrath K.A. (1975) TENS in treatment of post-operative pain. *American Journal of Surgery*, **130**, 338–340.

Warfield C.A., Skein J.M. & Frank H.A. (1985) The effect of TENS on pain after thoracotomy. *Annals of Thoracic Surgery*, **39**, 462–465.

Acupuncture

Dimond E.G. (1971) Acupuncture anaesthesia. *Journal of the American Medical Association*, **218**, 1558–1563.

Leong R.J. & Chernow B. (1988) The effects of acupuncture on operative pain and the hormonal response to stress. *International Anaesthesiology Clinics*, **26**, 213–217.

7: Operations on the Lung

Carcinoma of the bronchus is the most common indication for resection of the lung in the UK and, when operable, is treated surgically by lobectomy or pneumonectomy. Careful preoperative assessment and staging should prevent unnecessary thoracotomy which carries a significant risk even if the tumour is inoperable because of the extent of local spread and lymph node involvement. Some benign tumours, congenital malformations or secondary deposits are excised by segmental or wedge resection. Fungal infection, parasitic disease, bronchiectasis and tuberculosis also warrant pulmonary resection in some circumstances, and open lung biopsy can be required to establish the diagnosis and provide histological evidence of the stage or severity of diffuse diseases of the lung such as fibrosing alveolitis, alveolar proteinosis, eosinophilic granuloma and some types of lymphomata.

LIMITED RESECTIONS

Segmental and wedge resection

Segmental resection involves dissection and removal of a discrete bronchopulmonary segment, whereas wedge resection entails excision of a diseased portion of the lung irrespective of bronchopulmonary anatomy. The latter is usually a short procedure whereas the former is more time-consuming and carries many of the hazards associated with lobectomy. Discrete tumours such as benign hamartomata can sometimes be enucleated without causing much damage to surrounding tissue but it is usually necessary to close raw surfaces of the lung by direct suture or by means of a stapling device. The majority of patients presenting for limited resection of this sort have little or no impairment of pulmonary function unless they also suffer from coincidental disease such as asthma or chronic bronchitis. Endotracheal intubation is satisfactory and there are no particular constraints on the choice or management of the anaesthetic apart from recognizing that the operation is usually short.

Open lung biopsy

Transbronchial biopsy through the fibreoptic bronchoscope provides sufficient tissue for the diagnosis of diffuse lung disease in many patients. In the case of fibrosing alveolitis, however, several non-invasive techniques have now come to the fore in providing information concerning the presence, extent and progression of the disease. Broncho-alveolar lavage via the fibreoptic bronchoscope, high resolution computerized tomography (CT) and technetium-99m diethylene triamine pentacetic acid (^{99m}Tc DTPA) lung scanning can now be used to detect and characterize fibrosing alveolitis when symptoms are relatively minor and even when the chest radiograph is normal. Changes seen on high resolution CT may be pathognomic of many interstitial lung diseases and therefore there are now fewer indications for open lung biopsy. Sometimes, however, it is necessary to obtain a tissue specimen using open lung biopsy; this is particularly indicated if negative or equivocal findings have been obtained from other non-invasive investigations. Many of these patients are moderately or severely dyspnoeic, some are hypoxaemic at rest, and a restrictive defect with impaired gas transfer is the usual finding on formal lung function testing. Systemic corticosteroids and cyclophosphamide are used to treat some of these conditions and, occasionally, patients with presumed fibrosing alveolitis who are unresponsive to this regime will be treated with prednisolone and azathioprine. Particular care is therefore required to avoid introducing infection into the lungs or pleural space. The white cell and platelet counts should be checked preoperatively in patients receiving immunosuppressants or penicillamine, and it is customary, although probably not always necessary, to prescribe a steroid supplement with premedication for those currently or recently receiving corticosteroids.

Although the surgical procedure is minor, there is a notable morbidity and even mortality with fatality rates varying between 0.5 and 4.5% in reported series. The hazards are virtually always a reflection of the underlying disease or its treatment that complicate the postoperative rather than the operative period. It is usually possible to eliminate arterial hypoxaemia during surgery provided endotracheal rather than endobronchial intubation is chosen and an inspired oxygen concentration of 50% or more is used throughout. Unlike patients with airflow limitation, there is no tendency to sudden change in pulmonary function and few patients have excessive secretions within the respiratory tract.

Anaesthetic implications

Open lung biopsy is a short operation and so heavy premedication or large doses of long-acting muscle relaxants should be avoided, particularly in patients with severely impaired pulmonary function. Modern short-acting non-depolarizing neuromuscular blockers are particularly suitable agents for this procedure. Preoxygenation before induction is a sensible precaution in those who are hypoxaemic but it is rarely necessary to use more than 50% oxygen during the operation to keep the arterial oxygen tension equal to or greater than its preoperative value.

The extent of interference with respiratory function is minimized if surgery is carried out through a small incision below the axilla, although an anterior approach is sometimes preferred. The axillary route allows major muscle groups to be separated rather than incised and, on the right, provides easy access to all three lobes so that one or more biopsies can be taken from representative sites. The raw surface of the lung is closed, either by suture or with a lung stapler.

Persistent air leak in the postoperative period is an uncommon but serious complication of open lung biopsy. It is probably more common in patients with extensive fibrosis or eosinophilic granuloma. The need for a long period of drainage to the pleural cavity increases the likelihood of infection and so careful surgical closure of the lung surface is essential. Haemothorax or pleural effusion are occasional complications, and chest infections develop easily in those with marked restriction (a vital capacity less than 20% of the predicted lower limit of normal), who are often unable to cough effectively after operation. Most of these patients hyperventilate so that the arterial carbon dioxide tension is below normal, and high concentrations of oxygen can be given postoperatively without risk.

Patients who are severely dyspnoeic preoperatively, with a marked restrictive defect and severe arterial hypoxaemia, may benefit from a period of mechanical ventilation postoperatively. These patients are, however, in a very high-risk category and may be difficult to wean from ventilation unless specific therapy, based on the histological findings, improves their pulmonary function.

LOBECTOMY

Lobectomy is sometimes a straightforward operation which can be completed swiftly without need for blood transfusion. Conversely, extensive dissection and considerable haemorrhage are likely if there are many pleural adhesions, if tumour has infiltrated the chest wall or mediastinum, or when there has been longstanding infection and fibrosis.

It is desirable to isolate the operated lung for thoracotomy in the lateral position so that exposure is as good as possible and secretions can be controlled if necessary. An endobronchial blocker is theoretically ideal when secretions are confined to the resected lobe as may be the case in bronchiectasis (see implications of lobectomy for specific conditions, p. 156), but in the vast majority of cases intubation with a double-lumen endobronchial tube is satisfactory, even though it affords no protection against contamination of the remaining lobe on the operated side. The double-lumen tube provides access for suction to both lungs throughout, inflation or deflation of the operated lung to assist the surgeon whenever necessary, and easy re-inflation of the remaining lobe when the procedure has been completed. An unacceptable degree of arterial hypoxaemia occurs occasionally during one-lung anaesthesia in those with generalized pulmonary or bronchial disease who are, nevertheless, judged capable of withstanding lobectomy. Both lungs should be ventilated throughout in these circumstances but, once again, a double-lumen tube is useful because it provides independent access for suction to both lungs and so helps to limit the spread of secretions.

When the lobe has been isolated and the vessels clamped, ligated or sutured, and divided, the bronchus is cleared of adventitia, clamped and divided. The lobe is then removed. A bronchial stapler can be used to clamp and close the bronchus simultaneously. Alternatively, non-absorbable sutures are used to close the stump before the clamp is released and only in exceptional circumstances is it necessary to suture an open, unclamped bronchus. If this does prove necessary, it is convenient to be able to restrict ventilation to the non-operated lung only, even though it is generally possible to close the bronchus before the inevitable hypoventilation causes anxiety if only an endotracheal tube is in use.

The residual lobe is re-inflated after the bronchus has been closed. The integrity of the bronchial suture line is tested by pouring warm saline or water into the pleural cavity to cover the stump while a positive pressure of 30–40 cmH$_2$O is held by manual compression of the rebreathing bag. Some gas usually escapes during this manoeuvre, but it is generally from the raw surface of the lung left when the lobes have been separated and not from the bronchial stump.

Patchy collapse tends to recur in the remaining lobe while the drains are being inserted and haemostasis secured. These areas should be re-expanded before the chest is closed and the drains should be connected to the underwater seal as soon as the chest has been closed, preferably with suction applied too (Fig. 7.1). Careful endobronchial toilet is necessary before extubation and it is usually worth returning the patient to the supine position and ventilating by hand for a few breaths before removing the tube. Some surgeons like to carry out bronchoscopy after lobectomy so that secretions can be cleared from the remaining lobe under direct vision but this can be both difficult and traumatic in a partially paralysed and only lightly anaesthetized subject. Endobronchial suction carries less risk of causing serious hypoxaemia and is probably equally satisfactory, especially if it can be carried out through the two sides of a double-lumen tube.

Lobectomy and sleeve resection

An upper lobe can be removed with a circumferential cuff of the parent bronchus and continuity to the remaining lobe or lobes restored by an end-to-end anastomosis. This operation is indicated for bronchial neoplasms which involve the lobar bronchus so close to its origin that it cannot be divided from the main bronchus through healthy tissue. Endobronchial intubation of the contralateral main bronchus is preferred because it allows unhurried trimming and suturing of the two ends of the divided bronchus which are always of unequal diameter. A double-lumen tube without a carinal hook is satisfactory for this purpose. The endobronchial tube is very close to the open operative site during this type of surgery and so the introduction of infection is, at least in theory, a greater hazard than when the bronchus is divided distal to a sterile clamp. Passage of any endobronchial tube through the mouth precludes absolute sterility but all endobronchial apparatus, including the lubricant used on the bronchoscope and tube, should be sterilized before use and handled as little as possible.

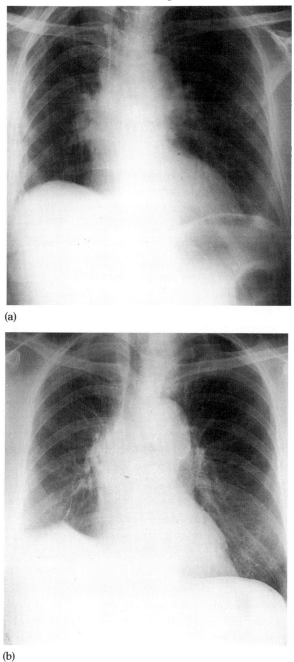

(a)

(b)

Fig. 7.1 Progress after uncomplicated right upper lobectomy. (a) Day one, a single apical drain remains. (b) Ten days later.

Implications of lobectomy for specific conditions

Bronchial neoplasms

Bronchial carcinoma is the most common overtly malignant primary tumour of the lung. Bronchial adenoma is less common and at one time was thought to be entirely benign. Many are locally invasive, however, especially the cylindromatous type which usually occurs in the larger bronchi and trachea. The other type of adenoma, the bronchial carcinoid, is a vascular tumour which is less often malignant and may extend into the bronchus as an endobronchial polyp. Some adenomata can be removed by bronchotomy and local excision but malignant tumours require resection of a lobe at least. Hilar lymph glands draining the resected lobe are always removed at the same time. The right middle and lower lobes are removed together if tumour or malignant glands involve their common bronchus.

It is rare for the neoplasm to cause much distortion of bronchial anatomy and endobronchial intubation with a double-lumen tube is usually straight-forward. If distortion is a problem a fibreoptic bronchoscope can be used to guide the double-lumen tube into position under direct vision (Chapter 5). Secretions retained beyond an obstructed bronchus or necrotic material from a cavitating squamous carcinoma are sometimes released during surgery (see Figs 5.3 and 5.4) but spread of disease is less of a problem by comparison with lobectomy for chronic suppurative disease. Haemorrhage during and after operation can be troublesome, especially if a peripheral tumour has infil-trated the chest wall, but is much less common than during or after pneumonectomy. Patients with the myasthenic syndrome complicating small-cell lung cancer rarely present for resection as they are usually inoperable at presentation; the anaesthetic implications of their management are discussed in Chapter 10, however. The other non-metastatic extrapul-monary manifestations of bronchial carcinoma such as hypertrophic pulmo-nary osteoarthropathy, endocrine disturbances, and the non-myasthenic neuromyopathies are very rare in patients suitable for resection.

Bronchiectasis

Patients with bronchiectasis can often be maintained in good health for years with regular postural drainage and antibiotics for infective exacerbations. There is a reluctance to advise resection because the disease is rarely localized to only one lobe, although some sites are more seriously affected than others. Infection is not necessarily eradicated by resection and may spread with time so that pulmonary function, often compromised at the outset, deteriorates even further. Some patients with localized disease are selected for surgery, however, especially if they suffer repeated haemoptyses or if infection is particularly difficult to control.

Careful preoperative assessment is essential and involves regional studies of structure (CT scanning and bronchography, Chapters 2 and 3) and sometimes of function (Chapter 2). Admission to hospital several days preoperatively should be arranged so that postural drainage, physiotherapy and antibiotics can reduce the volume and purulence of the sputum as far as possible. Many patients with bronchiectasis have variable airway obstruction and achieve better drainage of infected secretions if treated with bronchodilators. Corticosteroids are needed occasionally to relieve airway obstruction and, in spite of the vulnerability to infection which their use entails, purulent secretions can sometimes be cleared on steroids when drainage and antibiotics alone have failed.

A double-lumen tube is invaluable during resection for bronchiectasis because endobronchial suction is needed frequently and there are sometimes repeated requests for re-inflation of the lung to define tissue planes. There may be some distortion of the bronchial anatomy because of the longstanding fibrosis which accompanies chronic infection but it is usually basal and rarely sufficient to cause serious difficulty with endobronchial intubation.

The remaining lobe on the operated side is unprotected from the spread of secretions when a double-lumen tube is used, and infected material sometimes seeps past the endobronchial cuff into the opposite lung. Repeated suction using a sterile suction catheter each time limits this contamination and it rarely causes serious trouble postoperatively, provided physiotherapy and antibiotics are reinstituted immediately. The incidence of complications after lobectomy for bronchiectasis tends to be higher than after resection for uncomplicated carcinoma but is kept to the minimum by meticulous attention to sputum clearance and antibiotic treatment. If spread of secretions from lobe to lobe is likely to be a significant problem during lobectomy for bronchiectasis then bronchial blockade should be considered. We use a Fogarty embolectomy catheter to block selective bronchi during surgery for bronchiectasis and continue to ventilate the remaining lobes intraoperatively via an endotracheal tube. The use of bronchial blockers is discussed in Chapter 5.

Very occasionally, haemoptysis complicating bronchiectasis requires surgical treatment when resection is impossible because pulmonary function is too poor and the disease too widespread. Ligation of the bronchial artery supplying the bleeding area will often stop the haemoptysis but is only used as a last resort when treatment aimed at controlling infection has failed, and embolization of the bronchial vessels under radiological control has also been unsuccessful. Both lungs should be ventilated during anaesthesia but a double-lumen tube prevents haemorrhage from one side contaminating the other. The degree of surgical interference is usually minimal and most patients will breathe satisfactorily again immediately afterwards. If not, the double-lumen tube should be changed for an endotracheal tube and mechanical ventilation continued, although it is rarely needed for more than a few hours.

Tuberculous and fungal infections of the lung

Resection is rarely required in either of these conditions although an isolated tuberculoma, often undiagnosed preoperatively, is sometimes removed by wedge or segmental resection. A lobe or even a lung may require resection when destroyed by bronchiectasis which was originally tuberculous in origin, and active tuberculosis is occasionally treated surgically in patients with localized disease who default from treatment or are infected with *Mycobacterium tuberculosis* resistant to chemotherapy. There are theoretical grounds for interference between some of the anti-tuberculous drugs and anaesthetic agents but these are of no consequence in practice. It is far more important to ensure that chemotherapy is used to cover the operative period, that all anaesthetic apparatus is carefully sterilized after use, and that the selection and dose of anaesthetic drugs take account of factors such as cachexia or chronic alcoholism.

Cavitating pulmonary tuberculosis is often the antecedent for the development of an aspergilloma, i.e. chronic infection of a cavity, usually at the apex of the lung, with *Aspergillus fumigatus* (Fig. 7.2). Characteristically the mycetoma or ball of mycelia is visible on X-ray surrounded by a crescentric air space where the fungal mass is not attached to the walls of the cavity. Haemoptysis is a common and dangerous complication, usually provoked by additional bacterial infection, often with anaerobic organisms.

Antifungal chemotherapy is of little value but conservative treatment with antibiotics to control the bacterial pathogens is usually favoured initially because these patients generally have poor pulmonary function. In addition, surgical treatment carries a very high incidence of operative and postoperative complications, chiefly haemorrhage, septicaemia, persistent air leaks and bronchopleural fistulae. Some form of resection or drainage of the infected cavity is indicated, however, if haemoptysis is recurrent and life-threatening, or if bacterial infection cannot be controlled. If resection is

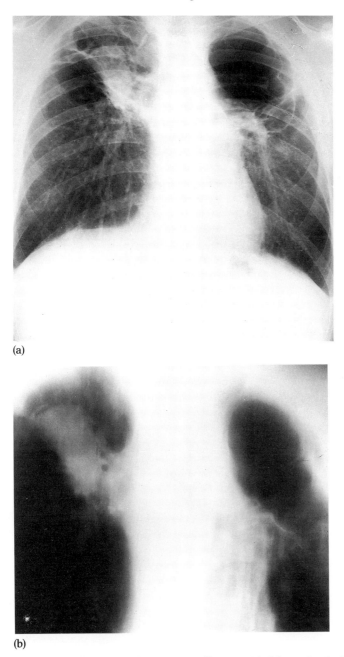

(a)

(b)

Fig. 7.2 (a) Postero-anterior view of pulmonary fibrosis with bilateral apical cavities. An aspergilloma had been removed from the left 2 years previously but there is another cavity on the right. (b) Single cut from a series of apical tomograms.

planned, the bronchus should be clamped early to help limit the spread of infection.

These patients are always difficult to manage. They are often debilitated because of chronic infection, and their pulmonary function is so poor that respiratory insufficiency can be precipitated by quite minor disturbances. They should be premedicated lightly, or given no premedication apart from atropine if operation is needed while there is active bleeding from the cavity. Endobronchial intubation can be difficult because apical fibrosis causes quite marked distortion of the carina and main bronchi. If this is so, a double-lumen endobronchial tube can be placed under direct vision using a fibreoptic bronchoscope. Alternatively selective bronchial blockade can be employed.

The postoperative period is likely to be stormy whatever surgical procedure is attempted: haemorrhage, infection and respiratory insufficiency are all common and require treatment along the usual lines. Mechanical ventilation is needed postoperatively in a proportion of these patients in spite of the chances of accentuating an air leak through the damaged lung.

Lobectomy after previous resection

A few patients require lobectomy months or years after an initial resection. This can be removal of the lobe remaining on the side of the first operation (completion pneumonectomy) or lobectomy on the side which was previously intact. Most of the implications of such an operation reflect the condition for which further surgery is indicated, but it must be remembered that functional pneumonectomy is the result whichever side is operated on. The other important consideration is that endobronchial intubation is almost always difficult because of the distortion caused by the first operation. It is often impossible to introduce a double-lumen tube blindly and, in these circumstances, the fibreoptic bronchoscope is an invaluable aid to the accurate placement of endobronchial tubes.

Complications of lobectomy

Patchy atelectasis, sputum retention and infection in the remaining lobe are quite common but usually respond well to physiotherapy, with antibiotics if necessary. The diaphragm rises on the operated side postoperatively and the remaining lobe, if healthy, will expand to fill the space in the majority of patients — especially if suction is applied to the chest drains. Failure of the remaining lobe to fill the pleural cavity is the most important complication of lobectomy and usually results in an apical air space, the accumulation of a pleural effusion and, often, a persistent air leak. Infection and bronchopleural fistula, although rare, are both much more likely in these circumstances. Occasional patients develop postoperative respiratory insufficiency, usually as a result of a combination of factors including preoperative pulmonary disease, sputum retention, or infection in the pleural space, remaining lobe or opposite lung. Mechanical ventilation is sometimes necessary and, although this increases the chance of a bronchopleural fistula developing or persisting, the hazards are far less than after pneumonectomy.

PNEUMONECTOMY

The usual indication for pneumonectomy is carcinoma of the bronchus and, although the results are not good, surgical treatment of squamous and adenocarcinoma carries a better 5 year survival rate at present than radiotherapy, particularly for adenocarcinoma which is relatively radioresistant. The management of oat cell (small cell, undifferentiated) carcinoma is more controversial, although here too there is renewed interest in resection when feasible, provided there is no evidence of extrathoracic spread.

Pneumonectomy cannot be advised lightly; it carries an overall mortality of up to 5% (UK Thoracic Surgical Register 1985–1987) with a higher mortality associated with right pneumonectomy. The explanation for the difference in mortality between right and left pneumonectomy is probably because the right lung is larger than the left (55% compared to 45%) and the incidence of bronchopleural fistula is higher after right pneumonectomy because the bronchial stump is less well protected than on the other side. Apart from operative complications such as haemorrhage, infection and the formation of a bronchopleural fistula, there is a significant morbidity and mortality because of the inevitable reduction in pulmonary function postoperatively. Criteria for selecting patients suitable for pneumonectomy are considered in Chapter 2.

Anaesthetic implications

Good preoperative preparation is essential and it is particularly important to familiarize the patient with the manoeuvres which will be required during postoperative physiotherapy. The practice of digitalizing patients prior to pneumonectomy has largely been discontinued (see Dysrhythmias, p. 113). The operation is carried out with the patient in the lateral position and a double-lumen tube is used to separate both lungs and provide one-lung ventilation when required. It is easy to test the integrity of the bronchial suture line if a double-lumen tube is used because it is only necessary to release the clamp on the lumen to the operated side before gradually applying an inflation pressure of up to 40 cmH$_2$O with the bronchial stump covered with water or saline.

One or two practical points are worthy of note during pneumonectomy. The incidence of dysrhythmias is higher than during lobectomy because there is more manipulation around the mediastinum. This is particularly true if the pulmonary veins are ligated within the pericardium in patients whose neoplasm is very close to the hilum. There is a small but definite risk of massive haemorrhage if clamps or ligatures slip from a pulmonary artery or vein, and it is important to prevent the patient coughing or straining while the vessels are being secured. Blood loss should be replaced generously because a considerable volume is lost with the specimen and further loss is likely to occur postoperatively as the space fills with fluid. The implications of closing and testing the bronchial stump are discussed above. Some surgeons choose to protect the bronchial stump, even at the time of primary resection, by dissecting an intercostal muscle bundle from the chest wall and suturing it, still supplied by its own vascular pedicle, over the closed surface of the bronchus. This step is, however, considered unnecessary by the majority of contemporary surgeons.

Once haemostasis has been secured, the chest is closed in the usual way but the principles of drainage differ from those which apply when functioning lung is left within the pleural cavity. The pleural space will fill with serosanguinous fluid after pneumonectomy and this should be allowed to accumulate, provided there are no postoperative complications and the mediastinum is not displaced to the non-operated side. This objective can be achieved if the chest is closed without drainage, especially if the mediastinum is centralized by aspiration of air immediately after the procedure, as described in the section on chest drainage in Chapter 6.

Closing the chest without drainage makes it more difficult to recognize serious postoperative haemorrhage. The possible hazard of introducing infection by inserting a drain is accepted by those surgeons who prefer to see the nature of the fluid which is accumulating, and to keep the space fairly empty for the first 24 hours. A single basal chest drain is used and is joined to an underwater seal bottle *without suction* (see also Chapter 6). It is left unclamped until the patient is lying on his or her back and breathing spontaneously. Some air usually escapes through the drain when the patient is turned from the lateral to the supine position, or if coughing occurs when spontaneous ventilation is being re-established; this should be allowed to escape so that the pressure does not build up within the space and cause surgical emphysema around the drain or the wound site. The mediastinum should be central at the end of operation if this routine is followed and, once this has been confirmed, the tube is clamped and remains so while the patient is returned for postoperative supervision. Thereafter it is unclamped for 1–2 minutes every hour for the first 12–24 hours so that the volume and nature of the drainage can be noted and any build up of pressure in the space avoided. It is usually possible to remove the drain on the first postoperative day when the risk of serious bleeding has passed.

Completion pneumonectomy and pleuropneumonectomy

Occasionally a completion pneumonectomy is undertaken in a patient who has undergone previous surgery such as lobectomy. Pleuropneumonectomy may also be undertaken in patients with a completely destroyed lung. In both these cases the tracheobronchial anatomy is often distorted so that endo-bronchial intubation may be difficult (Fig. 7.3). In the past we have achieved endobronchial intubation in this situation with a single-lumen tube placed under direct vision as there is no necessity to ventilate the diseased lung. Single-lumen tubes are no longer available so in future we are likely to use a disposable double-lumen endobronchial tube, sited in the healthy lung with the aid of the fibreoptic bronchoscope.

Both completion pneumonectomy and pleuropneumonectomy are likely to be difficult and long surgical procedures. Blood loss is often substantial and it may be necessary to continue intermittent positive pressure ventilation postoperatively via an endotracheal tube. This will allow the patient to rewarm and stabilize haemodynamically in the intensive care unit before spontaneous respiration is re-established.

Postoperative management

The pneumonectomy space gradually fills with a serosanguinous exudate and, unless the cavity has been drained, the fluid level reaches the upper border of the fourth thoracic vertebra by 48 hours and gradually fills the rest of the space more slowly thereafter (Fig. 7.4). Fibrinous bands develop quite rapidly so that the fluid is soon loculated and, given time, it fibroses. The diaphragm rises on the operated side and eventually fibrosis draws the mediastinum towards the side of resection so that the space is obliterated and there is progressive compensatory enlargement of the opposite lung.

The pneumonectomized patient should be sat up as soon as possible after operation to encourage expansion of the remaining lung. If turned into the lateral position, the operated side should remain dependent, so that the

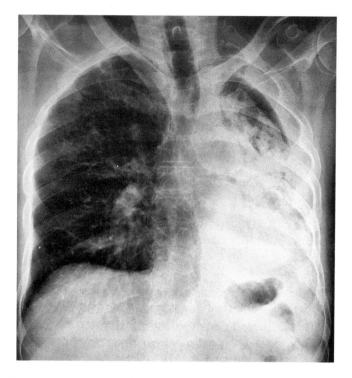

Fig. 7.3 Chest X-ray showing a left lung totally destroyed by tuberculosis, with apical cavitation. Pleuropneumonectomy was undertaken in this patient and endobronchial intubation was achieved with a disposable double-lumen tube sited under direct vision with the fibreoptic bronchoscope. Blood loss at surgery was in excess of 3 litres.

healthy lung is not compressed and there is little chance of fluid in the pleural space spilling into the trachea or bronchus on the opposite side. Humidified, oxygen-enriched air should be given by facemask throughout the first 12–24 hours and may be needed for longer in those with poor respiratory function.

Complications of pneumonectomy

Haemorrhage

Serious haemorrhage is more common after pneumonectomy than after lobectomy. Catastrophic bleeding results if ligatures slip off a pulmonary artery or vein, and can only be remedied by urgent re-operation. More gradual bleeding occurs because: a large surface is left around the cavity;

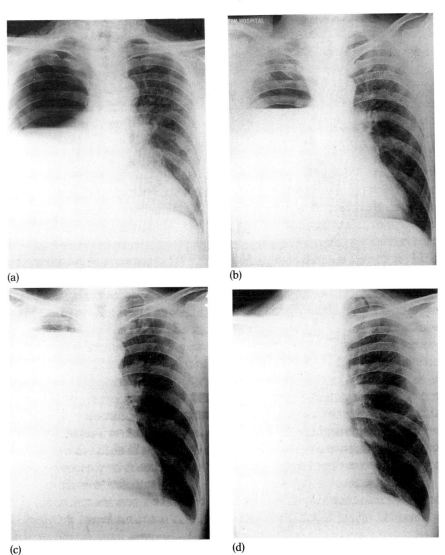

(a)   (b)

(c)   (d)

Fig. 7.4 Progress after uncomplicated right pneumonectomy. The space had been drained as described for 24 hours. (a) 48 hours after operation, (b) 2 weeks later, (c) 2 months later, (d) 4 months after operation.

vascular pleural adhesions may have been divided if the lung was adherent preoperatively; and extensive mediastinal dissection damages bronchial and mediastinal arteries. Postoperative haemostasis is favoured after lobectomy by the apposition of the remaining lobe against the chest wall but this safeguard does not apply after pneumonectomy. Volume replacement should be continued to replace known blood loss and should also allow for the blood and serous fluid which will accumulate within the space.

Excessive accumulation of fluid in the pneumonectomy space

Hypovolaemia and respiratory distress are the twin sequelae when the pneumonectomy space fills too rapidly and pressure builds up within it. Superficial vasoconstriction, sweating and oliguria are usual but the venous pressure is often misleading because it is likely to be high as a result of disturbances of intrathoracic pressure rather than low because of the reduction in blood volume. Right heart strain secondary to the reduction in area of the pulmonary vascular bed, together with pulmonary vasoconstriction caused by hypoxia, may also contribute. Tachycardia, a third heart sound and râles at the base of the remaining lung are common, and analysis of arterial blood reveals hypoxaemia with hypocarbia. It is very easy for this combination of symptoms and signs to be misinterpreted as sputum retention or left ventricular failure, but the condition is not an indication for more vigorous physiotherapy or for mechanical ventilation. Treatment with diuretics is ineffective and merely serves to deplete the already small circulating volume even further. Prompt relief usually follows drainage of the space but re-operation to evacuate haematoma may be necessary if the haemothorax has clotted. Once the excessive pressure in the space has been relieved, it is often clear that transfusion is also required to restore the depleted circulating volume. A similar syndrome occurring more insidiously 2–5 days postoperatively usually represents the accumulation of serous fluid and can be relieved by tube drainage or aspiration. Cardiorespiratory distress can also result if the space fills too slowly so that the mediastinum is displaced too far to the operated side. This unusual complication can be corrected by introducing air into the thorax on the side of surgery.

Displacement of the heart through an open pericardium into the pleural cavity after pneumonectomy is a rare complication, sometimes described as herniation of the heart. It is particularly dangerous on the right because the heart is not only displaced but also rotates on a pedicle formed by the great vessels, thus abruptly curtailing the return of blood to the ventricles or even obstructing it entirely. This emergency presents as sudden cardiovascular collapse with a very high venous pressure as a notable feature. It is rapidly fatal unless recognized and corrected immediately by re-opening the chest, in the ward if necessary. The presentation and sequelae are much less dramatic if herniation occurs on the left side.

Sputum retention, infection and respiratory failure

The risks of infection in the remaining lung are minimized by good preoperative preparation, protection of the remaining lung during surgery by endobronchial intubation, and adequate postoperative analgesia and physiotherapy. Appropriate antibiotic therapy and intensified physiotherapy form the basis of treatment if postoperative infection does occur. Some patients may not be able to clear secretions efficiently, particularly if a recurrent laryngeal nerve has been damaged, and this group will benefit from a mini-tracheotomy placed through the crico-thyroid membrane. This allows unhindered and effective bronchial toilet and in the majority of situations obviates the need for formal tracheostomy or mechanical ventilation. A proportion of patients develop respiratory insufficiency despite all these measures and, although mechanical ventilation following pneumonectomy carries a significant mortality, it must not be withheld if respiratory function is deteriorating rapidly and the patient is becoming distressed. The implications of mechanical ventilation in those with a suspected or proven broncho-pleural fistula are discussed on p. 170.

Infection of the pneumonectomy space causes an empyema and this may be the cause or the sequel of a small bronchopleural fistula. Drainage of empyema is discussed in Chapter 8, and the management of bronchopleural fistula is considered in detail on p. 168.

Dysrhythmias and pericarditis

A notable incidence of dysrhythmias, usually atrial in origin, is associated with pneumonectomy and they usually occur in the postoperative period. Their aetiology is obscure but may be related to surgical manipulation of the mediastinum, hypoxia, changes in vagal tone, or mediastinal displacement. The incidence of atrial dysrhythmias is lessened by preoperative digitalization which also curtails the rise in ventricular rate and consequent fall in cardiac output if atrial fibrillation (the most common rhythm disturbance) does occur. Prophylactic preoperative digitalization is not generally undertaken, however, although some surgeons commence digitalization at pneumonectomy if extensive mediastinal dissection proves necessary (see also Chapter 6 for a discussion on the treatment of postoperative dysrhythmias following lung resection). Direct current cardioversion or drug therapy postoperatively may be needed too, but cardioversion in particular is avoided if possible because the dysrhythmia may well recur and the hazards of treatment are greater in patients who are likely to be hypoxaemic. Electrocardiogram (ECG) signs of pericarditis are common after radical pneumonectomy, which involves securing the pulmonary veins within the pericardial sac, and should not be confused with postoperative myocardial infarction.

Miscellaneous complications

Renal failure is a recognized complication of any major operation and pneumonectomy is no exception. Hypoxia during or after operation can be an important contributory factor, as well as a reduction in cardiac output caused by hypovolaemia, abrupt reduction in the size of the pulmonary vascular bed, or distortion of the heart. Retention of urine is also common after major surgery and it may be necessary to catheterize the bladder to distinguish this from renal impairment.

Unexpected collapse is usually listed among the causes of death in series reporting pneumonectomy. Myocardial infarction, pulmonary embolism, ventricular tachycardia or fibrillation, and massive haemorrhage are all possible causes, and unrecognized severe hypoxaemia in a patient who is anaemic postoperatively can also be responsible.

Paraplegia is an extremely rare complication of thoracotomy and is usually attributed to damage to the spinal branches of intercostal arteries by imprudent dissection or diathermy at the posterior end of a rib.

BRONCHOPLEURAL FISTULA

This is one of the most dreaded, but rare, complications of pneumonectomy. Although an uncommon occurrence it is a favourite topic of examiners, possibly because its management encompasses a number of principles involving airway management. The term bronchopleural fistula refers to any communication between the tracheobronchial tree and pleural cavity and can result from trauma or neoplasm in the proximal bronchial tree, rupture of an inflammatory lesion or cavity within the lung into the pleura, or dehiscence of the bronchial stump after lobectomy or pneumonectomy. The symptoms and signs are variable and depend upon the size of the communication, the presence or absence of a chest drain, and whether or not there is fluid of any sort within the pleural space. Management of a fistula complicating an inflammatory or cavitating lesion in the lung is usually conservative and consists of drainage to the pleural space and antibiotics to control infection. Similar measures are usually all that is required for bronchopleural fistula after lobectomy, although occasionally surgical closure is necessary. Bronchopleural fistula as a result of injuries to the trachea and main bronchi is discussed in Chapter 9 and the rest of this section is devoted to bronchopleural fistula complicating pneumonectomy.

Factors which predispose to the formation of a bronchopleural fistula after pneumonectomy are: infection; residual neoplasm at the site of closure; the presence of a long or avascular stump; and poor surgical technique. The incidence of bronchopleural fistula following pneumonectomy is now extremely low in most units and is practically zero in the hands of one surgeon operating in the author's hospital. Surgical technique in closing the bronchial stump does appear to be a very important aetiological factor in the occurrence of bronchopleural fistula but there is generally no difference in the incidence of this complication between surgeons who suture the bronchial stump and those who staple it. If a surgeon has a high incidence of bronchopleural fistula with a suturing technique, however, he or she may well achieve better results by changing to a stapling device.

The fistula can present at any time, even many years after operation, but is most common within the first 3–14 days. The symptoms are unobtrusive at first if the fistula is small — little more than a low grade fever, slight tachycardia, and a persistent irritating cough with expectoration of small amounts of sputum which is almost always blood stained. Episodes of coughing at night and bouts of wheezy dyspnoea are particularly suggestive. An X-ray at this stage may either show a decrease in the volume of fluid in the space with an increase in the amount of air at the apex, or, the fluid level fails to go on rising as it normally does. Confirmation that a fistula is present can be obtained either by injecting methylene blue or radio-opaque contrast into the space and watching its appearance in the sputum or proximal bronchial tree, or by demonstrating that the space will not sustain a positive or negative pressure when air is injected or withdrawn from it. Sometimes a small fistula can be visualized at bronchoscopy when fluid from the space can be seen welling up through the stump, and it may heal if cauterized with sodium hydroxide or if sealed with a fibrin tissue glue. Even without cauterization, a significant proportion of small fistulae after pneumonectomy will heal without further intervention provided infection is controlled and the patient nursed so that fluid in the space is always below the level of the stump. Some clinicians feel that repeated aspiration of the pneumonectomy space will eliminate the chance of fluid spilling in significant quantities into the tracheobronchial tree, and is less likely to cause infection than a drain left in place continuously. This view is not held by others, however, who advocate drainage of the space in the presence of a significant but small bronchopleural fistula.

A large bronchopleural fistula after pneumonectomy presents dramatically although it is often preceded by a period of malaise, low grade fever, cough and haemoptysis as described above. This is followed by the abrupt onset of severe dyspnoea, usually after a bout of coughing and often precipitated by a change of posture which allows the operated side to be uppermost. Thin brown fluid which is characteristic of the contents of the space is both expectorated and inhaled into the remaining lung. It is often infected and always irritant so that it provokes bronchoconstriction and local inflammation causing severe respiratory distress and hypoxaemia. Signs of circulatory failure are usual too, probably caused by hypoxaemia but with septicaemia contributing as well in some cases. The diagnosis is usually clear on clinical grounds alone but can be confused with acute myocardial infarction or pulmonary embolism. If confirmation is required, chest X-ray will show a considerable fall in the fluid level in the pneumonectomized space and consolidation and collapse in the remaining lung (Fig. 7.5).

Prompt resuscitation is essential. The patient is sat up and supported so that the pneumonectomized side is dependent. Oxygen is given by facemask and it is wise to set up an intravenous infusion so that specific measures to control infection or treat dysrhythmias can be instituted if necessary. A chest drain should be inserted as soon as possible so that any fluid remaining in the space is removed and the risk of further contamination of the opposite lung is avoided. Postural drainage and physiotherapy have no place in the management of bronchopleural fistula of this magnitude but occasional patients require mechanical ventilation as part of resuscitation. When this is so, it is essential to use all the precautions described in the section on closure of bronchopleural fistula (see p. 173), and to isolate the fistula by using a single- or double-lumen endobronchial tube. Surgical closure of a fistula of this size is almost always necessary and is indicated as a matter of some urgency if intubation and mechanical ventilation are necessary because no type of endobronchial tube can be left in place safely for any length of time. A double-lumen tube may cause damage to the carina and so predispose to an increase in the size of the fistula. As discussed in Chapter 5, disposable double-lumen tubes tend to move *in situ* and are therefore very difficult to manage for long-term ventilation; and a single-lumen endobronchial tube is likely to kink during nursing manoeuvres.

Anaesthetic implications

Surgery may be needed before there is time for anything other than initial resuscitation but careful preoperative assessment is always essential, although this is likely to be mainly on clinical grounds. Particular attention-

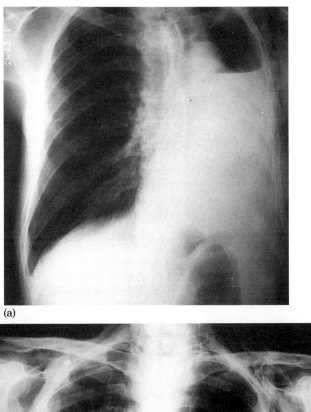

(a)

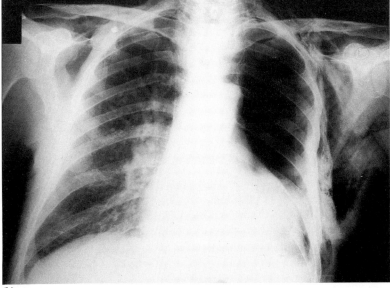

(b)

Fig. 7.5 (a) Postero-anterior chest X-ray of a 59-year-old man 10 days after left pneumonectomy. (b) Chest X-ray 3 days following that of Fig. 7.5a. Note almost complete loss of fluid in the pneumonectomy space and patchy consolidation in the right lung.

should be given to the degree of interference with pulmonary function, whether the circulation is stable or there are signs of poor peripheral perfusion, and the reported condition of the patient before the crisis. Evidence of infection may have been present for several days and some degree of malnutrition and dehydration is common.

The hazards associated with emergency anaesthesia in a patient who has been ill for some days after major surgery and who is suffering from uncontrolled or poorly controlled infection are all well known. Two other risks are specific to closure of the fistula. The first is that there is only one lung which is already damaged by the aspiration of the contents of the space from the opposite side. Any further contamination could result in asphyxia. The second specific hazard is that there is a route for air to escape from the tracheobronchial tree so that ventilation with positive pressure will, at best, be inefficient. If air enters the pneumonectomy space but cannot escape from it through the drain, the pressure which develops within the cavity will help to displace more of the contents of the space into the remaining lung. Pressurizing the chest by coughing has the same effect.

The requirements of the anaesthetic technique are that further hypoxaemia must be avoided at all costs, that entry of more fluid from the space into the lung must be prevented and that intermittent positive pressure ventilation (IPPV) should be withheld until the fistula has been isolated.

Endobronchial intubation under local anaesthesia is theoretically attractive because spontaneous ventilation and the ability to cough are retained until IPPV can be instituted safely. Similar advantages can be claimed for an inhalational general anaesthetic which is deepened to the point where intubation can be achieved without muscle relaxants.

These attractions disappear in practice. Local anaesthesia is difficult to use in a hypoxic, sick patient who may be unable to cooperate and who will cough when the spray or solution is applied. Penetration to the mucosa will be impaired if there are viscid or purulent secretions in the tracheobronchial tree and, if absorption is rapid, toxic reactions are more likely in those who are sick. Deep inhalational anaesthesia is equally unsatisfactory. The patient must be kept upright until intubated and so hypotension is likely with most commonly used inhalational agents such as halothane, enflurane and isoflurane. Spontaneous ventilation often fails before the depth of anaesthesia is sufficient to allow endobronchial intubation without coughing and may cease even before there is sufficient relaxation for easy laryngoscopy.

Preoxygenation followed by an intravenous induction and complete relaxation achieved with suxamethonium provides perfect conditions for atraumatic endobronchial intubation, with no risk of coughing or straining, but is only safe if the tube can be sited correctly and reliably at the first attempt. This is the method chosen by most experienced anaesthetists.

A single-lumen tube placed under direct vision into the remaining main bronchus was formerly recommended for isolating a bronchopleural fistula. A more modern, and equally effective approach, is to place a disposable double-lumen tube into the lung opposite the side of the fistula with the aid of the fibreoptic bronchoscope. The tracheal lumen on the pneumonecto-mized side is occluded before IPPV is begun to prevent pressure building up within the space.

Anaesthetic management

Most patients are not premedicated or given atropine alone but a small dose of a sedative is acceptable in those operated on for the closure of a small fistula in whom conservative management has failed.

During transfer to the operating theatre, the patient should remain sitting upright with the pneumonectomized side dependent. If possible the drain should be left unclamped but below the level of the patient for the journey. It is important to check that the drain remains unclamped before induction of anaesthesia. Full monitoring should be established from the outset. This will include an ECG, pulse oximetry and invasive arterial pressure monitoring. A reliable intravenous infusion is established, if this is not already in place, and it may be prudent to insert a central venous line under local anaesthetic. Suction apparatus, endobronchial equipment and drugs which may be required for resuscitation are checked at the beginning. It is safer to anaesthetize the most seriously ill patients in the operating room so that movement and disturbance after induction can be kept to a minimum.

The patient is induced and intubated while still sitting upright with the pneumonectomized side dependent; this is quite easy provided the anaes-thetist stands on a stool behind the head at the top of the table. Preoxygen-ation is followed by a sleep dose of suitable intravenous agent, such as etomidate, and then a fully paralysing dose of suxamethonium is adminis-tered. In some circumstances the surgeon will wish to bronchoscope the patient prior to intubation in order to inspect the fistula and suction the remaining lung. Once the lung has been cleared of secretions, Venturi ventilation can usually be achieved in the normal way.

Following bronchoscopy a suitable disposable double-lumen tube (usually the same size as used for the original operation) can be inserted into the larynx and positioned in the appropriate bronchus using the fibreoptic bronchoscope. If intubation proves difficult the rigid bronchoscope is re-inserted and Venturi ventilation continued whilst the situation is reassessed.

Once the double-lumen tube is in position the bronchial cuff is inflated and IPPV commenced to the remaining lung. The tracheal cuff is also inflated to aid stability of the tube. Once the fistula is isolated a non-depolarizing muscle relaxant is administered and an inhalational agent introduced to the inspired gas mixture. The patient is then lowered to the supine position and endobronchial toilet completed without hurry. Following this the patient is turned into the lateral position so the chest can be re-explored. It is essential that the endobronchial tube is not allowed to move during this latter manoeuvre.

Bleeding from the chest wall or pleural cavity is unusual and, unless there has been very extensive contamination of the remaining lung before intu-bation or the patient is particularly frail, the rest of the procedure is uneventful. It is usually possible to refashion and resuture the bronchial stump.

Spontaneous ventilation should be re-established at the conclusion of the operation if at all possible to avoid applying pressure to the recently closed stump and to eliminate the risk of further trauma when suction catheters are passed. If this proves impossible, ventilation should be continued through an endotracheal rather than an endobronchial tube for the reasons outlined previously, and the inspiratory pattern adjusted to provide a low peak inflation pressure. Theoretically, high frequency jet ventilation is preferable to conventional mechanical ventilation in these circumstances.

High frequency jet ventilation and bronchopleural fistula

High frequency jet ventilation (HFJV) has been advocated in the management of patients with bronchopleural fistula. This mode of ventilation is attractive because it does not necessitate endobronchial intubation and can provide satisfactory gas exchange with low peak inflation pressures. Mean airway pressures may be higher with some HFJV systems, however, when compared with conventional IPPV and this, combined with increased minute ventilation and higher flow rates, may lead to a greater flow of gas through a bronchopleural fistula (Fig. 7.6). Animal studies carried out to quantitate the effect of HFJV on the air leak through a bronchopleural fistula have produced conflicting results (see Further Reading).

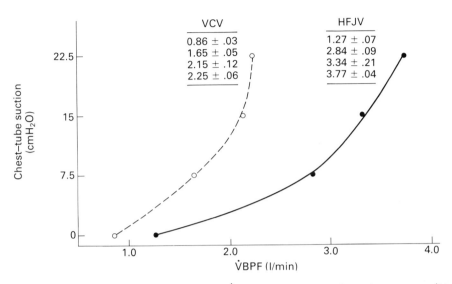

Fig. 7.6 Bronchopleural fistula flow rate ($\dot{V}$BPF) as a function of ventilator type and level of chest-tube suction. HFJV, high frequency jet ventilation; VCV, volume controlled ventilation. Flow was greater during HFJV at all levels of chest-tube suction. Reproduced with permission from Roth *et al.* (1988).

CYSTS, BULLAE AND LUNG ABSCESS

The terms cyst and bulla are often used interchangeably to refer to a thin-walled, air-filled cavity within the lung (Fig. 7.7) which is large enough to be seen on a plain X-ray. Isolated cysts are often congenital; acquired cysts are often multiple and may be a consequence of infection (e.g. staphylococcal pneumonia) or of degenerative disease such as emphysema. Congenital lobar emphysema (Fig. 7.8) is a rare condition, usually presenting in infancy, in which a single lobe is replaced by multiple air-filled cysts.

Cysts must have some communication with the bronchial tree, albeit often very small, otherwise the gas within them would be absorbed and the walls would collapse. Small cysts rarely cause any difficulty during anaesthesia or IPPV, although the chance of rupture and pneumothorax is higher than if they are not present, particularly if there is widespread disease of the lungs and airways as in emphysema.

A single large cyst in a patient with otherwise healthy lungs does not necessarily cause symptoms. However, it may enlarge and so compress surrounding tissue and displace the mediastinum if its communication with

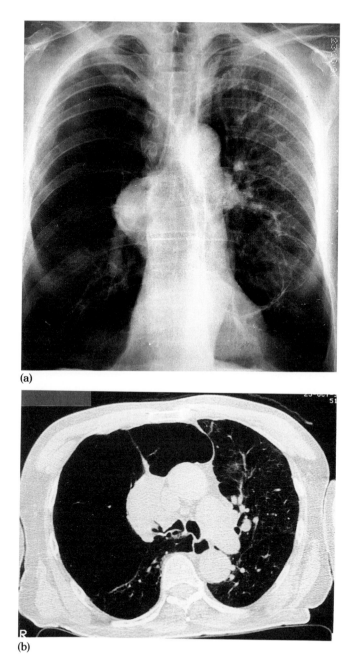

Fig. 7.7 (a) Chest X-ray showing gross cystic areas in right lung. (b) CT scan confirms cystic area with lack of lung markings on the right.

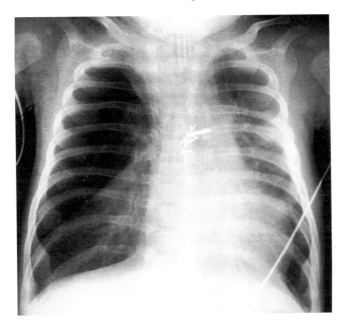

Fig. 7.8 Chest X-ray of a neonate with right middle lobe emphysema. The patient had previously undergone surgical repair of coarctation of the aorta and banding of the pulmonary artery. Resection of the diseased lobe was carried out with endotracheal anaesthesia.

the bronchial tree is valvular. A pneumothorax results if the cyst ruptures and this too is likely to develop tension because the communication with the bronchial tree is still present, especially when this is valvular in nature. Cysts of this type sometimes present in infancy, the usual manifestation being respiratory distress and reluctance to feed. Abrupt deterioration suggests that the cyst has ruptured. The features of congenital lobar emphysema are similar although there is usually less respiratory distress and less distortion of the mediastinum.

It is much more difficult to assess the significance of a large cyst or bulla in a patient with generalized emphysema in whom other abnormally large air-filled spaces are often also present. When the cyst is compressing surrounding lung tissue, pulmonary function may be improved and dyspnoea lessened if the cyst is removed. However, the risks of operation are high and recurrence is common, or a new cyst may develop elsewhere. Detailed studies of regional pulmonary function are desirable before removal of such cysts can be advised, and the best results are obtained if the rest of the lung tissue is reasonably healthy.

Anaesthetic implications of large lung cysts or bullae

The presence of a large air-filled cyst can never be ignored during anaesthesia, whether it is an isolated feature in a symptomless patient or merely
the largest of several cysts in a breathless patient with bullous emphysema.
The cyst is likely to enlarge whenever nitrous oxide is used because the
uptake of this soluble gas is faster than the clearance of less soluble nitrogen.
Any enlargement of the cyst can cause respiratory distress, and favours
rupture and the creation of a pneumothorax. It may be inflated preferentially
if mechanical ventilation is used, so causing inefficient gas exchange elsewhere and, if the communication with the airway is valvular, mechanical
ventilation is likely to make the cyst enlarge rapidly. These hazards apply
during anaesthesia for any form of surgery but, provided they are recognized,
it is usually possible to employ the conventional anaesthetic technique for the
procedure in question without disastrous consequences. Local anaesthesia is
obviously useful if suitable, and most anaesthetists would choose to avoid
nitrous oxide if general anaesthesia is essential. Spontaneous respiration
should be preserved, if it is safe to do so on other grounds, and the pattern
of mechanical ventilation should be adjusted to minimize the peak inflation
pressure, if controlled respiration is essential. Facilities for prompt drainage
of the pleural space or even of the cyst itself should be readily available. It
is impractical to attempt endobronchial intubation for emergency surgery in
patients who may have a full stomach, because of the possibility of aspiration
during a procedure which is more difficult and more time-consuming than
endotracheal intubation.

Gradual enlargement of the cyst may not be detected but rupture is
signified by the fairly sudden onset of respiratory distress, often accompanied
by the appearance or accentuation of bronchospasm. There is always a
marked resistance to inflation and usually signs of mediastinal displacement.
The presence of surgical drapes often makes auscultation of the lungs
impossible but the catastrophe cannot be left untreated until the conclusion
of the operation, and interference with surgery may be necessary. A chest
drain should be inserted and attached to an underwater seal bottle without
suction. A brisk air leak is likely to result but usually does not interfere with
adequate ventilation to the rest of the lung. Occasionally the cyst itself
enlarges to the point where respiratory distress occurs and this cannot be
distinguished on clinical grounds (or even sometimes on X-ray) from a
pneumothorax. Then there is no alternative to draining the cyst itself even
though this inevitably creates a large bronchopleural fistula. Here too,
however, satisfactory ventilation can usually be continued although the air
leak is likely to persist and surgical closure may well be necessary ultimately.

Thoracotomy for resection of lung cysts or bullae

Surgery is usually only advised to plicate and obliterate the cyst when it is already large enough to interfere with pulmonary function. Even a small increase in its size during anaesthesia may be dangerous in these circumstances, particularly if the rest of the lung is also abnormal. It could be argued that spontaneous ventilation should be preserved and nitrous oxide avoided until the chest has been opened so that the cyst and air leak can be controlled. Conversely, however, spontaneous ventilation is likely to be inefficient, especially in those most at risk who have widespread emphysema. Intubation with a double-lumen tube immediately after paralysis and induction of anaesthesia is usually the safest course. This permits ventilation of one or both lungs according to the circumstances. If the cyst is very large and unilateral it may be safer to ventilate the contralateral lung only until the chest has been opened. In many instances bullous disease is bilateral, however, and therefore it is sensible to ventilate both lungs initially, employing the lowest possible inflation pressure and omitting nitrous oxide from the inspired gas mixture. One-lung ventilation can then be used more safely, as requested, when the chest is open.

HFJV has been advocated for the intraoperative management of bullectomy and if both peak and mean airway pressures remain low this is a rational approach. Some jet ventilation systems produce an obligatory end-expiratory pressure, however, so pneumothorax remains a complication of their use.

In infants and children with lung cysts or lobar emphysema endobronchial intubation can be carried out with a single-lumen tube as briefly described in Chapter 5. Alternatively, a Fogarty embolectomy catheter can be used to block the main bronchus on the involved side. Endotracheal intubation and gentle manual ventilation with a gas mixture free of nitrous oxide is usually safe in practice, however, provided all the staff concerned are aware of the potential hazards.

Virtually all the risk associated with removal of lung cysts is over as soon as the chest has been opened and the surgeon is in a position to control the cyst. If problems with ventilation are anticipated, it is a wise precaution to delay induction of anaesthesia until monitoring apparatus and the intravenous infusion have been established, and the surgical team is scrubbed and ready to proceed immediately.

Intracavity drainage for bullous lung disease

Surgical excision of large bullae or cysts is a relatively major procedure and therefore less invasive intracavity drainage techniques have been developed to obliterate emphysematous bullae. A limited thoracotomy is performed and a small section of rib removed adjacent to the bulla. The pleura is then opened and the bulla incised. The interior of the bulla is inspected and any septa perforated prior to the insufflation of iodized talc into the space. A large Foley catheter is then inserted into the cavity via a separate stab incision in the chest wall. Purse string sutures are used to secure the Foley catheter within the bulla. Any free pleural space is also insufflated with talc, to obtain a postoperative pleurodesis, prior to insertion of a pleural drain and chest closure. Postoperatively the intrapleural drain remains on underwater seal suction until air leak ceases and the Foley catheter is connected to an underwater seal without suction for approximately 8 days. Initially there may be a large air leak from the bulla via the Foley catheter but this lessens as the bulla is decompressed and the space is gradually obliterated by the sclerosant effect of the talc.

Intracavity drainage techniques have been used in patients with a forced expired volume in 1 second (FEV_1) as low as 500 ml with a median improvement in this value of 22% postoperatively. However, those patients with an FEV_1 less than 500 ml and with a preoperative $Paco_2$ value above 7 kPa are unlikely to tolerate the procedure.

Endotracheal anaesthesia can be safely employed for the majority of patients undergoing intracavity drainage procedures provided an air/oxygen gas mixture is used and ventilation pressures are minimized. Adequate postoperative analgesia is essential to facilitate respiration but patients with marginal lung function may require a period of postoperative ventilation.

Fluid-filled cysts and cavities

Fluid-filled cavities (Fig. 7.9) are unlikely to increase in size during anaesthesia but are liable to rupture during manipulation so that the contents spill into the tracheobronchial tree. Theoretically, the lobe containing the cyst or abscess should be isolated with an endobronchial blocker but most anaesthetists would prefer to use a double-lumen tube which provides complete protection for the opposite lung as well as a route for suction to the bronchus on the operated side.

Most lung abscesses can be treated conservatively with antibiotics. They usually rupture into a bronchus and then postural drainage can be used to promote clearance and resolution. Occasionally the abscess ruptures into the pleural space; drainage to the pleural cavity is then needed and a bronchopleural fistula is likely to persist until the infection has been eradicated.

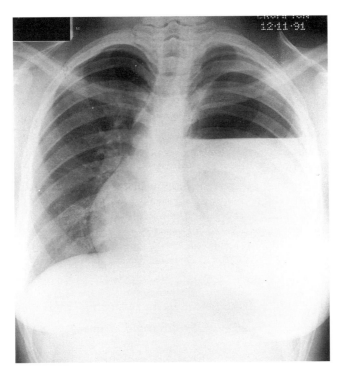

Fig. 7.9 Chest X-ray of a 14-year-old girl with a fluid-filled cavity in the left lung. This is an infected lung cyst which developed after surgery for the original, uncomplicated lung cyst had been refused.

Hydatid cysts

Hydatid disease is uncommon in most parts of the UK but is often seen in sheep-rearing countries. Without treatment, a hydatid cyst is likely to enlarge, form daughter cysts or rupture, though sometimes it merely dies and calcifies. Dissemination of the scolices, the infective larvae of the parasite, results in the formation of secondary cysts, and an acute anaphylactic reaction can occur if fluid from the cyst is absorbed into the systemic circulation. Regression of hydatid cysts after treatment with mebendazole has been reported but surgical removal is often necessary. Unlike pyogenic abscesses, hydatid disease is difficult to control with chemotherapy and so it is essential that the cyst is removed without spilling any of the infected contents. Lobectomy may be necessary to remove a large cyst or one which is secondarily infected with pyogenic bacteria, but small cysts can be enucleated and removed intact. Sometimes the cyst is aspirated and then injected with 10% formalin to kill the scolices and prevent dissemination if the cyst ruptures during removal. In addition, the whole operating field is draped with swabs soaked in formalin. Alternatively, a cryoprobe can be used to freeze a small area of the exposed cyst wall which is then incised and the contents evacuated. A 0.5% solution of silver nitrate (which is not toxic to healthy tissue but sterilizes scolices within 2 minutes) is then instilled into the empty cavity so that the rest of the wall can be removed without risk. It is unlikely, but possible, that a hydatid cyst will rupture into the airway during surgery and so some form of endobronchial intubation is advisable, generally a disposable double-lumen tube. Occasionally bilateral pulmonary hydatid cysts are removed at the same operation. A median sternotomy provides adequate access in some cases and causes less postoperative pain, but bilateral thoracotomy may be needed and warrants particular attention to pain relief (see Chapter 6).

FURTHER READING

Limited resections, open lung biopsy

Du Bois R.M. (1992) Management of fibrosing alveolitis. *British Journal of Hospital Medicine,* **47**, 680–683.
Macfarlane J. (1985) Lung biopsy. *British Medical Journal,* **290**, 97–98.

Lobectomy and pneumonectomy

Cassorala L. & Katz J. (1984) Management of cardiac herniation after intrapericardial pneumonectomy. *Anesthesiology,* **60**, 362–364.
Chattopadhyay D.K. (1979) Surgical treatment of bronchiectasis. *Annals of Royal College of Surgeons,* **61**, 195–197.
Goodman L.R. (1980) Post-operative chest radiograph II. Alterations after major intra-thoracic surgery. *American Journal of Roentgenology,* **134**, 803–813.
Key M. (1985) What it is like to lose a lung. *British Medical Journal,* **290**, 142–143.
Kirsh M.M., Rotman H. & Behrendt D.M. (1975) Complications of pulmonary resection. *Annals of Thoracic Surgery,* **20**, 215–235.
Spiro S.G. (1990) Management of lung cancer. *British Medical Journal,* **301**, 1287–1288.
Suarez J., Clagett O.T. & Brown A.L. (1969) The post-pneumonectomy space: factors influencing its obliteration. *Journal of Thoracic and Cardiovascular Surgery,* **57**, 539–542.
Verheijen-Breemhaar, L., Bogaard J.M., Van den Berg B. & Hilvering C. (1988) Post-pneumonectomy pulmonary oedema. *Thorax,* **43**, 323–326.

Bronchopleural fistula

Donnely J.A. & Webster R.E. (1991) Computer-controlled anaesthesia in the management of bronchopleural fistula. *Anaesthesia,* **46**, 383–384.
Feeley T.W., Keating D. & Nishimura T. (1988) Independent lung ventilation using high-frequency ventilation in the management of a bronchopleural fistula. *Anesthesiology,* **69**, 420–422.

Lauckner M.E., Beggs I. & Armstrong R.F. (1983) The radiological characteristics of bronchopleural fistula following pneumonectomy. *Anaesthesia*, **38**, 452–456.

Orlando R., Gluck E.H., Cohen M. & Mesogites C.G. (1988) Ultra-high-frequency jet ventilation in a bronchopleural fistula model. *Archives of Surgery*, **123**, 591–593.

Roth M.D., Wright J.W. & Bellamy P.E. (1988) Gas flow through a bronchopleural fistula. Measuring the effects of high-frequency jet ventilation and chest-tube suction. *Chest*, **93**, 210–213.

Ryder G.H., Short D.H. & Zeitlin G.L. (1965) The anaesthetic management of a bronchopleural fistula with the Robertshaw double-lumen tube. *British Journal of Anaesthesia*, **37**, 861–865.

Cysts, bullae and lobar emphysema

Benumof J.L. (1987) Sequential one-lung ventilation for bilateral bullectomy. *Anesthesiology*, **67**, 268–272.

Cote C.J. (1978) The anesthetic management of congenital lobar emphysema. *Anesthesiology*, **49**, 296–298.

Kan A.F. & Oh T.E. (1992) Anaesthesia for bullectomy. Use of propofol, high frequency jet ventilation and extradural blockade. *Anaesthesia*, **47**, 480–482.

Kinnear W.J.M. & Tattersfield A.E. (1990) Emphysematous bullae. Surgery is best for large bullae and moderately impaired lung function. Editorial. *British Medical Journal*, **300**, 208–209.

McCarthy G., Coppel D.L., Gibbons J.R. & Cosgrove J. (1987) High frequency jet ventilation for bilateral bullectomy. *Anaesthesia*, **42**, 411–414.

Morgan M.D.L., Edwards C.W., Morris J. & Matthews H.R. (1989) Origin and behaviour of emphysematous bullae. *Thorax*, **44**, 533–538.

Venn G.E., Williams P.R. & Goldstraw P. (1988) Intracavity drainage for bullous, emphysematous lung disease: experience with the Brompton technique. *Thorax*, **43**, 998–1002.

8: Operations on the Pleura, Chest Wall and Diaphragm

PLEURAL DISEASE

Pleurectomy and pleurodesis

The most common indication for pleurodesis or pleurectomy is to prevent the recurrence of spontaneous pneumothorax. Debulking pleurectomy is occasionally undertaken as a palliative procedure to prevent the recurrence of pleural effusions in mesothelioma and other malignant conditions. However, it is now more common to chronically drain persistent malignant effusions via a pleuroperitoneal shunt.

Spontaneous pneumothorax

Primary spontaneous pneumothorax usually occurs in young adults, more frequently in males, and with a much higher incidence in smokers. These patients are often tall and thin and it has been suggested that the occurrence of pneumothorax is related to the presence of a sharp posterior angle in the second rib. Tiny apical bullae, often multiple, are usually present in these otherwise healthy subjects, and pneumothoraces are often recurrent on the same or opposite side (Fig. 8.1). Secondary pneumothorax occurs most often in patients with chronic bronchitis and emphysema and is caused by the rupture of a subpleural bulla. Less frequently, pneumothorax is a complication of tuberculosis, lung abscess, cystic fibrosis or bronchogenic carcinoma.

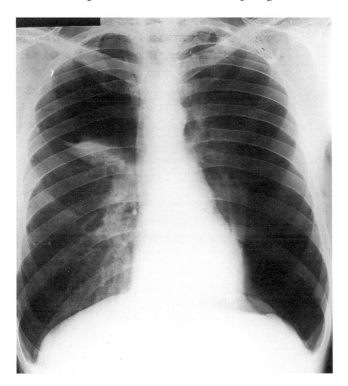

Fig. 8.1 Bilateral spontaneous pneumothoraces. The right lung has not collapsed completely because of adhesions after a previous pneumothorax. Right pleurectomy was carried out uneventfully after the left pleural cavity had been drained and the lung expanded. Left pleurectomy was carried out at a subsequent operation several months later.

A small pneumothorax will resolve without treatment but drainage allows a rapid and more certain re-expansion of the lung. A tension pneumothorax requires urgent chest drainage and it may be necessary to insert a large-bore needle through the chest wall, to relieve pressure as an emergency, before formal insertion of the chest drain. In the majority of cases there is enough time to confirm the diagnosis radiologically before inserting the drain, but care must be taken to differentiate pneumothorax from lung cysts, lobar emphysema, a dilated stomach after closed chest trauma causing diaphragmatic rupture or, very rarely, stomach or bowel herniated through a congenital defect of the diaphragm.

Chest drains are usually inserted through the fourth or fifth interspace in, or a little anterior to, the mid-axillary line. Here there is little in the way of muscle between skin and rib cage, and the tubing will lie to the side of a recumbent patient, so minimizing discomfort. This site of entry is furthest from the mediastinum, therefore lessening the chance of puncturing a major blood vessel, and is also preferred to the second interspace anteriorly for cosmetic reasons.

A healthy lung will re-expand quickly and fill the hemithorax as soon as the pleural cavity has been drained; apposition of the lung to the chest wall usually stops the leak of air although suction is often needed to promote re-expansion of the lung. Sudden re-expansion of a lung can, albeit very rarely, result in pulmonary oedema usually confined to the ipsilateral lung (Fig. 8.2). This is thought to be due to increased vascular permeability in the lung leading to exudation of protein-rich fluid into the alveoli.

Pleurectomy is indicated if the pneumothorax recurs, if there is a history of pneumothorax on the opposite side or, in some circumstances, as a prerequisite for employment after only one pneumothorax. Air leaks from the surface of a damaged lung are often persistent, especially in patients with emphysema, and the combination of immobility, pain from the drain, and the leak itself leads to a gradual deterioration in pulmonary function. Pleurodesis or pleurectomy are clearly hazardous but may be the only way to eradicate the leak.

Pleurectomy is carried out through an anterolateral thoracotomy; the parietal pleura is stripped over all but the diaphragmatic and mediastinal surfaces of the hemithorax and the incision also provides access to bullae or sites of air leakage which can be ligated at the same time. The pleural cavity is drained postoperatively and suction used to keep the lung fully expanded so that it adheres to the chest wall over a wide area. There is now an increasing trend towards endoscopic thoracic surgery and pleurectomy has been undertaken by this route. The long-term results and recurrence rate of pneumothorax following endoscopic pleurectomy are as yet unknown, however.

Physical pleurodesis — the abrasion of both pleural surfaces with a gauze swab — can be carried out through a much smaller incision. Alternatively, iodized talc can be insufflated during thoracoscopy or even, albeit less effectively, through a chest drain. This is a highly irritant substance which sets up an inflammatory reaction and so promotes the formation of pleural adhesions (Fig. 8.3). Although the procedure itself is less disturbing than pleurectomy, the chemical pleurisy which results is very painful; immobility and interference with respiration are inevitable and there is a definite morbidity and even mortality associated with pleurodesis in patients with severe underlying lung disease. Pleurectomy is more reliable as a means of preventing recurrence of the pneumothorax and treating its cause, and so is

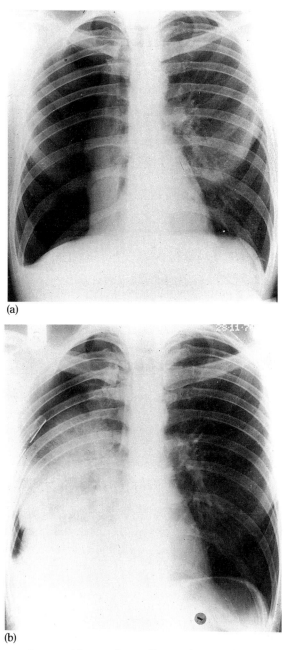

(a)

(b)

Fig. 8.2 (a) Pneumothorax with complete collapse of the right lung, which had probably been present for about a week at presentation. (b) 18 hours later when there is incomplete expansion and gross pulmonary oedema on the right.

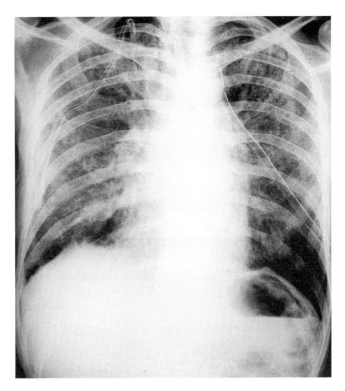

Fig. 8.3 Bilateral, widespread infiltration in a patient with Hodgkin's disease. Repeated pneumothoraces on both sides had necessitated bilateral drainage for a number of weeks. The air leaks were sealed by bilateral pleurodesis using talc insufflation.

preferred in all but the most debilitated patients. There has, however, been a trend towards more conservative treatment of recurrent pneumothorax in patients with cystic fibrosis. In those patients who might be future candidates for heart-lung transplantation, intercostal drainage, chemical pleurodesis, ligation of bullae, or limited surgical pleurodesis is carried out in preference to pleurectomy. This limits the problem of major haemorrhage encountered during heart-lung transplantation in patients who have had a previous pleurectomy.

Anaesthesia for pleurectomy or pleurodesis

Factors which should be considered at the preoperative visit include the size of any existing pneumothorax, whether or not it is drained effectively, the magnitude of air leaks through it, the state of the underlying lung and, above all, the condition of the lung on the opposite side. It is rarely possible or even desirable to obtain meaningful measurements of pulmonary function which require a forced expiratory manoeuvre, although recent information may be available in patients with longstanding disease who have been followed regularly. Patients with generalized lung disease may need a short period of mechanical ventilation postoperatively and those at risk should be warned in advance of this possibility. Every effort should be made, if time permits, to eradicate infection within the bronchial tree; this applies particularly to patients with cystic fibrosis in whom pneumothorax is often a complication of the later stages of the disease, when surgical treatment is hazardous.

Anaesthesia with nitrous oxide and mechanical ventilation in the presence of a pneumothorax is associated with several theoretical hazards which are largely eliminated if the pleural cavity is drained already. Some patients do present for surgery with a small, unresolved and undrained pneumothorax. This may enlarge during mechanical ventilation, can develop tension, or may increase in size as a result of the uptake of nitrous oxide. The interval between induction of anaesthesia and opening the pleural cavity is usually short however and, provided both anaesthetist and surgeon are aware of the potential problem, it is rarely necessary to take any special precautions. If in doubt, ventilation with an air/oxygen mixture rather than with nitrous oxide and oxygen should be considered. A double-lumen tube is not always necessary, although it provides better control if the air leak is large. A pneumothorax may occur during operation on the non-operated side and this is less likely if the tidal volume can be delivered to both lungs rather than one, so decreasing the airway pressure. When a double-lumen tube is in place it is preferable, therefore, to ventilate both lungs until one-lung anaesthesia is requested by the surgeon. Development of a pneumothorax on the non-operated side during any one-lung anaesthetic is a serious complication which should always be considered if there is progressive resistance to inflation accompanied by increasing hypoxia and signs of carbon dioxide retention. If this possibility is suspected, the surgeon may be able to confirm or refute the diagnosis by aspirating the opposite pleural cavity through the mediastinum. If a pneumothorax is confirmed on the opposite side, it is necessary to insert a chest drain before continuing with the operation, even if this does involve disturbance to the drapes.

Apart from the risks of pneumothorax, the only problems encountered during operation are likely to reflect underlying lung disease, for example, emphysema or cystic fibrosis. Haemorrhage is occasionally troublesome, particularly during resection of a mesothelioma where the tumour involves both visceral and parietal pleura and there are no clear planes of demarcation.

Bilateral pleurectomy is undertaken occasionally, preferably through a median sternotomy which not only provides access to both sides during one operation but also causes less postoperative pain and interference with respiratory function than bilateral thoracotomy. Continuous display of the arterial blood pressure is essential during this procedure because the heart and great vessels can be compressed and distorted while the surgeon is operating in one or other pleural cavity. Access and exposure for the surgeon are less satisfactory than if bilateral thoracotomy is chosen, and use of a double-lumen tube allows collapse of one or other lung if necessary.

It is usually both possible and desirable to re-establish spontaneous ventilation at the end of the operation but occasional patients with limited lung function require mechanical ventilation for a short period. So too may those with good lung function who have been subjected to a bilateral procedure, particularly if this has been carried out through separate thoracotomy incisions. Postoperative pain is severe after pleurectomy or pleurodesis and requires adequate treatment (see Chapter 6).

Insertion of a pleuroperitoneal shunt

Patients with a persistent malignant effusion can be palliated by chemical pleurodesis after drainage of the effusion, performed via a small thoracotomy, or alternatively a pleuroperitoneal shunt can be inserted. The former procedure is usually carried out when it is thought that the lung will expand to fill the chest and obliterate the pleural space. If the lung is unlikely to expand sufficiently then a shunt is inserted. The shunt drains pleural fluid into the peritoneum via a one-way valve which is inserted subcutaneously in the chest wall. The patient is asked to massage the valve mechanism at regular intervals in order to aid the forward flow of fluid.

Light general anaesthesia and paralysis, with ventilation via an endotracheal tube, are usually satisfactory for both the above procedures. Pleurodesis causes severe pain and should be treated appropriately in the postoperative period. The main concern to the anaesthetist is the preoperative state of the patient and the likely effect of the operation on respiratory function. Many of the patients will be dyspnoeic preoperatively and although one would expect an improvement in lung function when the effusion is drained this is not always the case. For example, tumour invasion of the thoracic cage causes a mechanical restriction to respiration and this may be exacerbated when the underlying diseased lung adheres to the chest wall following pleurodesis.

Drainage of empyema

An empyema or purulent effusion within the pleural space occurs most commonly as a complication of an inflammatory process in the underlying lung, for example, pneumonia, lung abscess, tuberculosis or an infected pulmonary infarct. Spontaneous rupture of the oesophagus, chest trauma and infection following thoracic surgery are other causes. Even if the empyema can be sterilized with antibiotics, the thick exudate will not absorb but will fibrose, so restricting movement of the lung on that side. Adequate drainage is essential therefore and, in the acute stage, is carried out by inserting an intercostal drain under local anaesthesia. Drainage may be incomplete if the fluid is locular or particularly thick, and the limited space between adjacent ribs restricts the size of tubing which can be inserted without causing local pain. Once the empyema is chronic and the lung is adherent, rib resection or even fenestration is necessary to achieve successful drainage.

An empyema is often associated with a bronchopleural fistula, particularly after pneumonectomy, and so it is preferable in the acute stages to insert the drain under local anaesthetic with the patient sitting upright. Much more extensive analgesia is required for rib resection; extensive infiltration is neither particularly safe nor reliable in the presence of infection, and so it is usually preferable to induce general anaesthesia for rib resection and drainage. This is providing that care is taken to isolate any existing or potential bronchopleural fistula using one of the techniques described in Chapter 5. Careful postoperative bronchial toilet and antibiotic cover are usually sufficient to control the spread of infection if the lung remaining on the side of surgery is contaminated while the empyema is being drained.

Fenestration is a more radical procedure which involves the removal of parts of three or four ribs so creating a large chronic drainage site. The procedure is unpleasant and was carried out under local anaesthesia in the past, but this is unnecessary, provided precautions are taken to isolate any bronchopleural fistula.

Decortication

A thick, fibrous layer forms around the lung as a result of infection, haemothorax or some types of uninfected inflammatory effusion; this may need to be removed surgically if the lung is to expand fully and move freely on that side. Decortication or removal of this fibrous layer is carried out through a thoracotomy which permits removal of fibrous tissue from both the visceral and parietal surfaces. It is often extremely difficult to identify tissue planes and therefore it is helpful to maintain ventilation to both lungs to assist the surgeon in identifying the edge of the lung and residual plaques of fibrous tissue. Sometimes it is difficult to re-expand a chronically collapsed lung and fill the hemithorax on that side; haemorrhage and air leaks from the surface of the lung are major intra- and postoperative complications. Occasionally, structures underlying the pleura such as the phrenic nerve, diaphragm or azygos vein are damaged during dissection.

Benign pleural thickening of either the visceral or parietal pleura can occur in the form of plaques or more extensively in one hemithorax. An appearance resembling a peripheral tumour is created if localized pleural fibrosis causes infolding of the underlying lung (Blesovsky syndrome); thoracotomy may be required to excise the visceral pleura and free the lung if the diagnosis is in doubt or if the patient presents with chest pain.

SURGERY ON THE CHEST WALL

Correction of sternal deformity

Pectus excavatum and pectus carinatum (pigeon chest) are the two main types of chest wall deformity presenting for surgery. Pectus excavatum is the more common and consists of a concavity of the anterior chest wall of varying severity, usually in the lower two-thirds of the sternum (Fig. 8.4). The physiological sequelae of the deformity are trivial although some patients have a vital capacity a little below the lower limit of predicted normal, and there is some evidence that cardiac function is impaired during severe exercise in the upright position. Correction is usually carried out to improve appearance but it is difficult to interpret the statement made by some patients that their exercise tolerance is impaired preoperatively and improved by surgery.

At operation, the sternum is mobilized and supported in its new position by a metal strut or bar which lies behind it. If necessary, the bar can be removed at a later date after the sternum has healed. Anaesthetic management is straightforward: mechanical ventilation through an endotracheal tube is entirely satisfactory and spontaneous ventilation can be re-established immediately afterwards. Haemorrhage and pneumothorax are occasional complications but in general the morbidity is extremely small. There is extensive dissection of costal cartilages during surgery and this causes severe postoperative pain if analgesia is inadequate. Epidural analgesia should be considered in this group of patients.

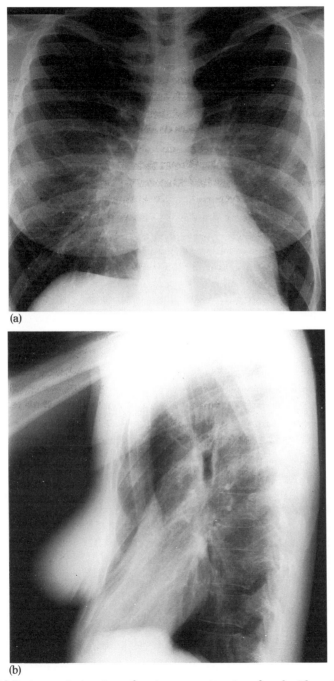

(a)

(b)

Fig. 8.4 (a) Postero-anterior view of pectus excavatum in a female. There is also a mild thoracic scoliosis. (b) Lateral view.

Stabilization of chest wall; resection of chest wall

The operative fixation of rib and sternal fractures is the treatment of choice in only a few centres. 'Internal splinting' by intermittent positive pressure ventilation (IPPV) is usually preferred if the chest wall is very unstable, if there are severe extrathoracic injuries, or if the patient is known to suffer from pre-existing pulmonary disease. Less severe injuries can be managed with local analgesia which allows the patient to breathe spontaneously, cough effectively and cooperate with physiotherapy. Serial measurements of the vital capacity are useful as a means of identifying patients who are unable to tolerate this conservative regime. Injuries to the chest wall are often associated with damage to the lung, airway, heart or great vessels. In addition, haemothorax and pneumothorax are both common and it is often necessary to drain the chest, especially if mechanical ventilation is to be used. The management of ruptured bronchus and traumatic rupture of the diaphragm is discussed elsewhere but other aspects of chest trauma are beyond the scope of this book.

Major resection of the chest wall is necessary occasionally in the treatment of malignant disease, and haemorrhage is the main intraoperative anxiety. Postoperative pain is severe and respiratory insufficiency is common, especially after resection of lung as well as chest wall. Resection of the posterior chest wall, particularly that covered by the scapula, does not lead to such instability that occurs when large areas of the anterior chest wall are excised. Gross paradoxical movement of the chest wall is likely to lead to respiratory failure and sputum retention in all but the very fit patient. The insertion of a chest wall prosthesis will ameliorate this situation but not eliminate it.

Intercostal arteries may be sacrificed at or near their origin during chest wall resection. Rarely this can compromise the blood supply to the anterior spinal artery causing neurological damage. In the past we have not used thoracic epidural analgesia with either local anaesthetic drugs or opoids after chest wall resection because of the additional risks of hypotension, epidural haematoma or direct damage to the cord. Adequate pain relief is, however, essential after this procedure to aid respiration and sputum clearance. We therefore now use lumbar or high-lumbar opioid epidural analgesia in the postoperative period after prior discussion with the patient and surgeon.

Thoracoplasty

Thoracoplasty was used extensively from the early 1930s until the mid-1950s to produce permanent collapse and healing of tuberculous cavities. A classical extrapleural thoracoplasty involved the resection of several ribs and was usually carried out in stages, often under paravertebral block. The availability of effective chemotherapy for tuberculosis has virtually eliminated the need for these extensive operations, but more limited thoracoplasties are still occasionally performed to obliterate chronically infected spaces such as chronic empyemata and bronchopleural fistula following upper lobectomy, or to close the infected space remaining as a result of previous collapse therapy. A limited thoracoplasty is sometimes performed at the same time as the initial resection if there is any doubt about the ability of the remaining lung to fill the hemithorax, for example, after resection of an aspergilloma.

The operation is painful and nowadays is carried out under general anaesthesia. Management is governed to a large extent by the nature of the disease for which thoracoplasty is indicated, but it should always be assumed that a bronchopleural fistula may be present or may develop intraoperatively,

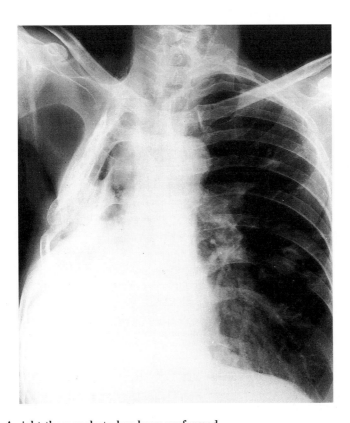

Fig. 8.5 A right thoracoplasty has been performed.

and that blood loss is likely to be considerable. Adequate pain relief is essential postoperatively and every effort must be made to secure maximum expansion of healthy lung on the side of the thoracoplasty. Paradoxical movement of the chest wall may be a problem after an extensive thora-coplasty, and it was this which led to the introduction of the staged procedure. Strapping a firm pad over the affected area of the chest wall is the traditional remedy but care must be taken to prevent this interfering with normal chest wall movement elsewhere (Fig. 8.5).

DIAPHRAGMATIC HERNIA

Trauma and major congenital defects are the usual causes of diaphragmatic hernia presenting for repair.

Congenital diaphragmatic hernia in the neonate

Neonates presenting with a large diaphragmatic hernia usually have a defect in the posterolateral part of the diaphragm (foramen of Bochdalek) — 80% of these occurring on the left. The majority of these babies require urgent surgery if they are to survive but some reach adult life with few symptoms, particularly if the hernia is small. An eventration of the diaphragm (Fig. 8.6) has much less serious consequences.

Respiratory distress is the main symptom of diaphragmatic hernia and many infants will require endotracheal intubation and resuscitation at birth. Intra- and extrauterine surgery on the foetus is just beginning to offer a therapeutic option before birth which may, to some extent, alleviate the long-term problems of pulmonary hypoplasia. This type of surgery is, however, in the early phases of development.

The diagnosis of diaphragmatic hernia is suggested by an empty, scaphoid abdomen; bowel sounds can be heard in the chest and an X-ray shows stomach and intestine in the thorax. The lung on the affected side is collapsed and usually hypoplastic, and the mediastinum is displaced to the opposite side. The opposite lung is usually hypoplastic too, although to a lesser degree. These babies should only be treated in centres familiar with the implications of major cardiothoracic surgery in the neonatal period and should be transferred after initial resuscitation. Surgery for neonatal diaphragmatic hernia was formerly considered an emergency but surgery does not correct the underlying pulmonary abnormality and respiratory function usually deteriorates immediately following operation. A policy of elective preopera-tive stabilization with optimization of ventilation and treatment of pulmonary

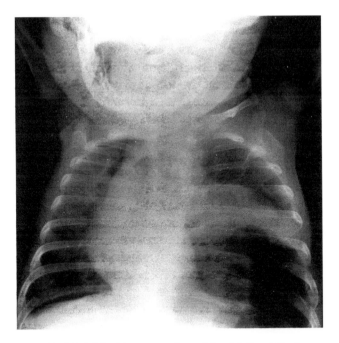

Fig. 8.6 A 4-month-old child with eventration of the left hemidiaphragm.

hypertension appears to offer the best chance of a successful outcome. Despite this, overall mortality rates of up to 30% are still reported.

In neonates with severe lung disease accompanying diaphragmatic hernia alternative methods of support such as high frequency jet ventilation (HFJV) and extracorporeal membrane oxygenation (ECMO) have been employed, particularly in North America. This treatment is complex and expensive and has yet to find widespread favour in European centres, although multicentre trials are planned for the near future.

Congenital diaphragmatic hernia in the adult

Occasionally a congenital hernia through the foramen of Bochdalek does not present until adult life. The usual symptoms are dyspnoea because the herniated abdominal contents compress the lung, and dyspepsia, colic, vomiting and haematemesis caused by obstruction and ulceration in the herniated stomach. The patient may present acutely with signs of intestinal obstruction and with bowel sounds audible in the chest. A chest X-ray confirms the diagnosis, provided herniation is distinguished from eventration

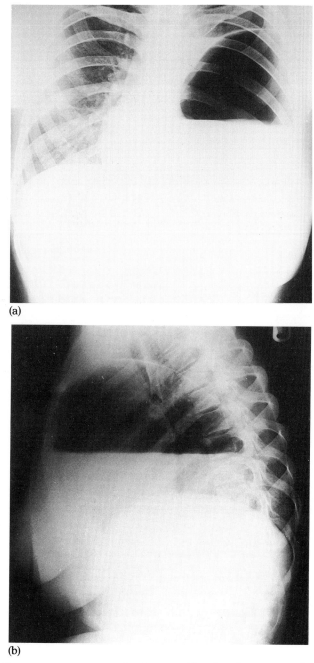

(a)

(b)

Fig. 8.7 (a) Postero-anterior view of a 19-year-old girl with a previously undiagnosed left diaphragmatic hernia. The stomach is dilated and contains a fluid level; it lies entirely within the chest. (b) Lateral view.

or elevation of an atrophied hemidiaphragm. If dyspnoea is the major presenting symptom and a large gas-filled stomach is present in the chest (Fig. 8.7), the condition can be mistaken for a spontaneous pneumothorax and a chest drain inserted with disastrous consequences.

Surgery for repair of an adult diaphragmatic hernia is undertaken through a thoracotomy but an abdominal incision may be necessary as well if necrotic bowel has to be resected. Electrolyte disturbances should be corrected preoperatively and a nasogastric tube should be passed to decompress the stomach. The abnormal position of the stomach means that reflux is more likely during induction of anaesthesia, and all precautions should be taken to prevent aspiration of gastric contents into the lungs, even if there is no clinical evidence of obstruction. One-lung anaesthesia is usually unnecessary if the condition is longstanding, but may be useful if an acute hernia is present as a result of trauma.

Traumatic diaphragmatic hernia

Diaphragmatic hernia can result from blunt or penetrating injuries; it may present acutely or remain asymptomatic for years, and sometimes follows apparently trivial trauma. Herniation is more common on the left side, presumably because the right diaphragm is protected by the liver. Repair of an uncomplicated traumatic hernia is carried out through the chest in much the same way as for the congenital condition, although the nature and extent of associated injuries will influence the management of patients requiring emergency surgery.

FURTHER READING

Pleural disease

Childress M.E., Moy G. & Mottram M. (1971) Unilateral pulmonary edema resulting from treatment of spontaneous pneumothorax. *American Review of Respiratory Diseases*, **104** 119–121.

Cohen J.D., Loewinger J., Zelikovski A. & Gassner S. (1991) Unilateral pulmonary oedema of the contralateral lung following transaxillary sympathectomy. *Anaesthesia*, **46**, 651–653.

Desiderio D.P., Meister M. & Bedford R.F. (1987) Intraoperative re-expansion pulmonary oedema. *Anesthesiology*, **67**, 821–823.

Fentiman I.S. (1987) Effective treatment of malignant pleural effusions. *British Journal of Hospital Medicine*, **37**, 421–428.

Firmin R.K. & Tolhurst Cleaver C. (1980) Safe intrapleural drainage. *Anaesthesia*, **35**, 79–80.

Harriss D.R. & Graham T.R. (1991) Management of intercostal drains. *British Journal of Hospital Medicine*, **45**, 383–386.

Hodson M.E. (1989) Managing adults with cystic fibrosis. Editorial. *British Medical Journal,* **298**, 471–472.

Lamberty J.M. & Rubin B.K. (1985) The management of anaesthesia for patients with cystic fibrosis. *Anaesthesia,* **40**, 448–450.

Morris V. & Wiggins J. (1992) Current management of pleural disease. *British Journal of Hospital Medicine,* **47**, 753–758.

Seddon D.J. & Hodson M.E. (1988) Surgical management of pneumothorax in cystic fibrosis. *Thorax,* **43**, 739–740.

Empyema

Goldstraw P. (1979) Treatment of post pneumonectomy empyema: the case for fenestration. *Thorax,* **34**, 740–745.

Goldstraw P. (1980) Post pneumonectomy empyema — the cloud with a silver lining. *Journal of Thoracic and Cardiovascular Surgery,* **79**, 851–855.

Surgery on the chest wall

Beiser G.D., Epstein S.E., Stampfler M., Goldstein R.E., Noland S.P. & Leuitsky S. (1972) Impairment of cardiac function in patients with pectus excavatum with improvement after operative correction. *New England Journal of Medicine,* **287**, 267–272.

Editorial (1977) Management of the stove-in chest with paradoxical movement. *British Medical Journal,* **1**, 1242.

Heydorn W.H., Zajtchuk R., Schuchmann G.F. & Strevey T.E. (1977) Surgical management of pectus deformities. *Annals of Thoracic Surgery,* **23**, 417–420.

McCoy J.A. & Ayim E. (1976) The management of acute thoracic injuries. *Anaesthesia,* **31**, 532–537.

Moore B.P. (1975) Operative stabilisation of non-penetrating chest injuries. *Annals of Thoracic Surgery,* **70**, 619–630.

Ravitch M.M. (1977) *Congenital Deformities of the Chest Wall and their Operative Correction.* W.B. Saunders, Philadelphia.

Weeden D. (1991) Management of thoracic trauma. In: Taylor I. & Johnson C.D. (eds) *Recent Advances in Surgery,* Vol. 14 pp. 198–214. Churchill Livingstone, Edinburgh.

Diaphragmatic hernia

Bray R.J. (1979) Congenital diaphragmatic hernia. *Anaesthesia,* **34**, 567–577.

Charlton A.J., Bruce J. & Davenport M. (1991) Timing of surgery in congenital diaphragmatic hernia. *Anaesthesia,* **46**, 820–823.

Chatrath R.R., El Shafie M. & Jones R.S. (1971) Fate of hypoplastic lungs after repair of congenital diaphragmatic hernia. *Archives of Disease in Childhood,* **46**, 633–635.

Ehrlich F.E. & Salzserg A.M. (1978) Pathophysiology and management of congenital posterolateral diaphragmatic hernias. *The American Surgeon,* **44**, 26–30.

Finer N.N. & Etches P.C. (1992) Timing of surgery in congenital diaphragmatic hernia. *Anaesthesia,* **47**, 536–537.

Harrison M.R. Bjardal R.I., Longmark F. *et al.* (1978) Congenital diaphragmatic hernia. The hidden mortality. *Journal of Pediatric Surgery,* **13**, 227–231.

Keiltz S.R. (1980) Congenital diaphragmatic hernia: 10 years' experience. *Anaesthesia,* **35**, 1136.

9: Operations on the Tracheobronchial Tree and Oesophagus

REMOVAL OF INHALED FOREIGN BODY

Foreign bodies are inhaled at any age but, most commonly, by children under the age of three. Acute upper airway obstruction is the immediate hazard; alternatively, the foreign body is inhaled deep into the tracheobronchial tree where it impacts, sets up a local inflammatory reaction which wedges it more securely in place, and ultimately causes distal collapse and infection. Inorganic objects such as fragments of poorly manufactured toys are also troublesome. Organic material is more dangerous because it swells after inhalation and may fragment, even before attempts are made to remove it. Peanuts are particularly liable to swell and fragment and they liberate an irritant oil which causes severe local inflammation. Sweets are a problem too because they dissolve in the tracheobronchial secretions, so forming a viscid, hypertonic solution which predisposes to obstruction and collapse.

A specific history of inhalation is only available in a proportion of cases and is often absent in children, or in adults after alcoholic excess, or dental surgery carried out under general anaesthesia but without endotracheal intubation. Paroxysmal cough and wheeze are the common presenting symptoms in children but dyspnoea, stridor, fever and vomiting also occur. A chest infection which fails to clear in spite of antibiotic treatment in an otherwise healthy child may warrant chest X-ray and diagnostic bronchoscopy to exclude the presence of an inhaled foreign body. In adults, a cavitating pneumonia, lung abscess or bronchiectatic area may be the consequence, although other obstructive lesions are more common in this age group.

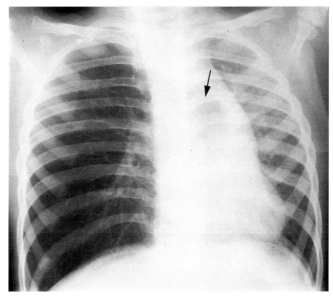

Fig. 9.1 Inhaled foreign body in a 6-year-old boy, acting as a ball-valve in the right main bronchus. The right lung is overdistended (arrowed), has displaced the mediastinum to the left and has extended anteriorly across it.

The majority of foreign bodies lodge in the right lung because of the disposition of the right main bronchus relative to the trachea, but approximately 20% are found on the opposite side. Radio-opaque material can sometimes be seen on a plain chest X-ray, and obstructive emphysema of a lobe or lung occurs if the foreign body acts as a ball-valve in a bronchus (Fig. 9.1). More often the radiological appearances are non-specific, with atelectasis and consolidation but no obvious bronchial lesion, or even no abnormality at all.

Rigid bronchoscopy to remove the foreign body should be carried out as soon as possible; a trial of postural drainage is not defensible. Bronchotomy or even lobectomy may be necessary if the foreign body is deeply embedded in a mass of inflammatory tissue or has eroded through the wall of the bronchus. Bronchial stricture is another consequence of delay in removal. The rigid bronchoscope is preferred to the fibreoptic instrument because it allows the passage of much larger instruments (and foreign bodies), and the open-ended rigid instrument also makes ventilation easier in small children.

Anaesthesia for removal of inhaled foreign body

The general principles governing anaesthesia for bronchoscopy are discussed in detail in Chapter 3. Particular difficulties which may be encountered during the removal of foreign bodies, especially in children, are that the airway is sometimes already compromised, the patient is unprepared, and infection in the lungs is often well established. Movement of the foreign body, short of complete removal, may cause or worsen respiratory obstruction, and laryngeal spasm or oedema can contribute too if the cords are traumatized by repeated passage of the bronchoscope. A selection of endotracheal tubes of varying sizes should be available, including several smaller than would normally be selected, together with facilities for tracheostomy. Spontaneous respiration should be preserved if there is upper airway obstruction. An inhalational induction (e.g. halothane in oxygen) will usually achieve a sufficient depth of anaesthesia for laryngoscopy to locate the foreign body. Very rarely, tracheostomy is necessary to secure the distal airway when removal of a proximal, obstructing foreign body proves difficult.

An inhalational induction, followed by deep general anaesthesia with spontaneous respiration throughout, is still chosen by some anaesthetists for the removal of foreign bodies from the respiratory tract in children. In the absence of upper airway obstruction light general anaesthesia with muscle relaxants is usually satisfactory and less traumatic. Anaesthesia is induced inhalationally, in the usual way, and then suxamethonium is administered via an indwelling venous cannula to facilitate rigid bronchoscopy. In adults and larger children without upper airway obstruction it is safe to use an intravenous induction. Once the bronchoscope has been passed through the cords, and there is no likelihood that the foreign body will be further displaced, ventilation can be commenced. As outlined in Chapter 3 a modern, ventilating paediatric bronchoscope (Figs 3.2 and 3.3) is the safest and most convenient way of ventilating a child during bronchoscopy. The child can be kept anaesthetized with an inhalational agent in a high inspired oxygen concentration whilst the foreign body is located and removed. Gentle manual ventilation will prevent fragments from being blown further into the lungs and the sole use of an inhalational agent will allow rapid awakening, even after a prolonged procedure. Ventilation will, necessarily, be intermittent as forceps are placed down the open-ended bronchoscope and therefore it is essential to monitor the electrocardiogram (ECG) and oxygen saturation. Intermittent suxamethonium can be used to provide muscle relaxation in children undergoing bronchoscopy but atropine should be available to give intravenously if bradycardia occurs. If the procedure is likely to be prolonged a short-acting non-depolarizing agent, such as atracurium or vecuronium, can be given once the airway has been secured.

A Venturi device can be used to ventilate children during bronchoscopy provided the size of needle matches the bronchoscope appropriately (see

Chapter 3). It should be possible to maintain adequate gas exchange without excessive inflation pressures, even when a small bronchoscope is in use. Care must be taken to avoid overinflation of the lungs when either an instrument or the foreign body is blocking the bronchoscope, and ventilation may need to be interrupted from time to time to prevent the foreign body or its fragments being blown deeper into the respiratory tract when they are loose within the bronchial lumen. In general, manual inflation via a T-piece circuit and ventilating bronchoscope is safer.

A large foreign body cannot be removed through a small bronchoscope and must therefore be grasped with forceps and extracted while the bronchoscope is withdrawn simultaneously. Repeated instrumentation may be necessary and, even in skilled hands, this will traumatize the vocal cords and upper respiratory tract. An alternative solution, which has been reported, is to pass a Fogarty embolectomy catheter beyond the foreign body; the balloon is inflated and the catheter withdrawn so that the foreign body is trapped against the tip of the bronchoscope and the entire assembly is removed together.

Postoperatively the patient should be supervised closely until fully conscious. Laryngeal stridor is relatively common, particularly after a difficult and prolonged procedure in a small child. These patients should be managed postoperatively in an intensive care unit and allowed to breathe humidified oxygen by facemask. Intravenous corticosteroids should be given if there is anxiety about laryngeal oedema, although immediate improvement cannot be expected. Endotracheal intubation, using a tube smaller than would be chosen normally, is necessary if there is severe stridor or signs of respiratory obstruction and after a long bronchoscopy it may be safer to allow the child to awaken with an endotracheal tube in place. Spontaneous respiration can be permitted through the tube in the majority of cases, and extubation undertaken as soon as there is an obvious free leak of gas around the tube when positive pressure is applied to the lungs. Facilities for immediate re-intubation should be available and occasional patients will require more prolonged intubation, or even mechanical ventilation, if an extensive pneumonia is established before the foreign body can be removed.

TRACHEAL RESECTION

Trauma, tracheostomy and prolonged endotracheal intubation are the usual causes of benign strictures requiring resection. Single or multiple papillomata occur very occasionally in the trachea and can usually be removed endoscopically. The cylindroma, or adenoid cystic carcinoma, is classified as an adenoma but, although it rarely metastasizes, it is locally invasive. It is more common in the trachea than the carcinoid type of bronchial adenoma and in this site is second in frequency only to a carcinoma.

The tracheal lumen must be markedly reduced before dyspnoea is a prominent symptom. An irritating, non-productive cough is a common feature of localized tracheal lesions, and a wheeze or stridor may be audible; this is sometimes influenced by posture and often misdiagnosed as asthma. Drugs used in the management of bronchial asthma are, in general, totally ineffective but corticosteroids are occasionally useful, particularly if mucosal oedema is contributing to the obstruction. Those with very severe obstruction usually obtain some relief by inhaling a mixture of helium and oxygen. This has a density far less than air and, under the turbulent flow conditions existing at the site of an incomplete obstruction in the upper respiratory tract, will pass the obstruction much more readily.

The severity of tracheal obstruction can be assessed clinically by means

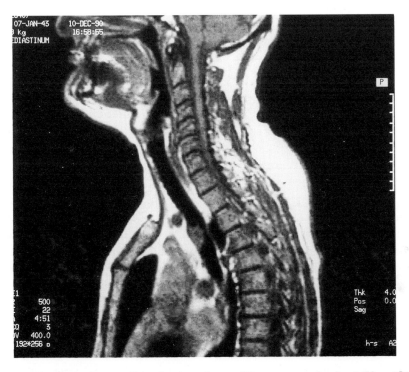

Fig. 9.2 MRI scan of the neck and upper thorax. Note tumour clearly visible within the trachea opposite the level of the manubrium. Reproduced with permission from J.W.W. Gothard, 1993.

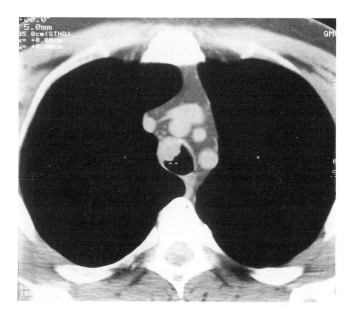

Fig. 9.3 CT scan of the same patient as in Fig. 9.2, clearly demonstrating the tracheal tumour in cross-section.

of the flow-volume loop (see Chapter 2), and also by a variety of imaging techniques. Plain X-rays and tomograms of the thoracic inlet are sometimes sufficient to define the site and extent of a stricture but a computerized tomography (CT) or magnetic resonance imaging (MRI) scan (see Chapter 2) is usually much more helpful (Figs 9.2 and 9.3).

Anaesthesia for tracheal resection

Tracheal resection is performed infrequently and, as it so clearly carries the risk of interfering with gas exchange, the details of intraoperative management should be discussed beforehand by the surgical and anaesthetic staff.

Operations on the upper trachea are carried out through a cervical incision but right thoracotomy is required for access to the lower trachea and carina. Gas exchange during the resection can be achieved by intubation of the lower trachea or a main bronchus through the surgical incision, or by ventilation with either a Venturi device or high frequency jet ventilation (HFJV), both delivering gases through a fine catheter which passes beyond the divided trachea. Extracorporeal circulation is an alternative for complicated resections, usually those involving the carina, but most surgeons prefer to avoid it because of the greater complexity and the far higher risks of operative and postoperative haemorrhage. The choice between jet ventilation and intermittent positive pressure ventilation (IPPV) through a cuffed endotracheal tube inserted through the incision depends upon the preferences of the staff concerned and on the location of the lesion.

Selection of equipment

Endotracheal tubes of greater than average length should be available in a range of sizes regarded as normal or small for the patient in question. Sterile anaesthetic tubing, connections and tubes are prepared if intubation of the distal trachea or main bronchi is planned during operation; a co-axial Bain circuit is popular in preference to conventional tubing because it occupies less space within the thoracotomy wound. Flexible, armoured endotracheal tubes are convenient because they can be manipulated or retracted easily by the surgeon without compromising the airway. However, many other patterns have been used or improvised successfully for individual circumstances. Sterile catheters, 8–10 French gauge (1.5–2 mm internal diameter) and approximately 12 in (30 cm) in length, are used if jet ventilation is chosen, although the size of catheter may have to be matched to a particular ventilation system.

Emergency equipment should always be available, including a paediatric bronchoscope and the instruments and tubing required for tracheostomy. The latter is only of value as a means of relieving obstruction caused by a stricture high in the trachea, and should be avoided if at all possible because of the risks of infection and of interfering with the mobility of the trachea.

Anaesthetic technique

Patients with marked respiratory obstruction should be premedicated lightly or not at all, but sedation is desirable in those with lesser degrees of obstruction because turbulent airflow is at a minimum during quiet respiration. An intravenous infusion, pulse oximetry and an ECG should be established before induction. Frequent or even continuous estimation of arterial blood gas tensions will also be required and it is useful to insert an arterial cannula under local anaesthesia at the same time so that the blood pressure can be displayed during intubation.

Preoxygenation followed by an intravenous induction with propofol and a short-acting muscle relaxant is satisfactory and safe for patients with a moderate obstruction who are only dyspnoeic on exercise. Once the airway has been secured a longer-acting neuromuscular blocker can be administered. Intubation under local anaesthesia may be preferred in those with a severe stenosis in whom there is doubt about the ease or even feasibility of intubation. Alternatively, an inhalational induction followed by intubation during spontaneous respiration can be considered. However, this will be time-consuming and it may be difficult to deepen the anaesthetic to the point where reflexes from the respiratory tract are abolished and muscle relaxation is sufficient for easy visualization of the larynx.

It is usually possible to site the endotracheal tube so that its tip lies above the tracheal lesion and the majority of patients can be ventilated satisfactorily through the stenosed segment (Fig. 9.4a). On the very rare occasions when this is impossible, a small endotracheal tube of greater than normal length may have to be passed through the stricture. However, it is preferable to pass a paediatric bronchoscope through the stenosis and use the injector technique to maintain ventilation until the trachea has been opened. In this way, intubation through the stricture is less likely to cause serious haemorrhage or push the tumour further down the respiratory tract. If the latter manoeuvre is necessary anaesthesia can be maintained with intravenous propofol, otherwise inhalational anaesthesia with the addition of a moderate dose of opioid is satisfactory.

Management of ventilation

Use of an endotracheal tube. The stricture is identified and the trachea mobilized for some distance above and below. It is transected below the stricture and a second, flexo-metallic armoured endotracheal tube is inserted into the distal segment by the surgeon (Fig. 9.4b). Mechanical ventilation is continued through sterile ventilator tubing attached to this second endotracheal tube, and the first tube is then withdrawn proximally but left with its tip between the vocal cords so that it can be advanced at a later stage. The stricture can then be resected and the posterior anastomosis between the upper and lower segments completed while the armoured tube is retracted laterally or forwards (Fig. 9.4c). There is usually no difficulty in mobilizing the trachea sufficiently to allow approximation of the cut ends, unless the stricture or tumour-bearing area is unusually long. The armoured endotracheal tube is withdrawn once the posterior wall has been reconstituted and then the original tube is advanced into the distal trachea with its tip guided through the partially completed anastomosis by the surgeon (Fig. 9.4d). Ventilation is continued through this tube while the anterior trachea is sutured. The endotracheal tube can be withdrawn into the upper

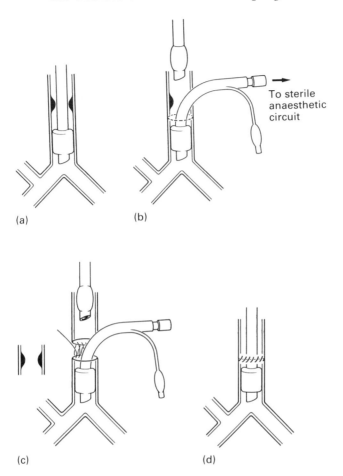

To sterile
anaesthetic
circuit

(a)

(b)

(c)

(d)

Fig. 9.4 (a) Small endotracheal tube passed beyond a tracheal tumour. (b) A sterile endotracheal tube is passed directly into the trachea distal to the tumour. The original tube is withdrawn but left through the larynx. (c) The tumour is excised and the posterior tracheal anastomosis fashioned as ventilation is continued via the second endotracheal tube placed directly into the distal trachea. (d) The second endotracheal tube is withdrawn to allow completion of the anterior anastomosis with the original tube in place.

trachea as soon as both tracheal suture lines have been completed, but this arrangement leaves the anastomosis exposed to positive pressure throughout the remainder of the operation and it may be preferable to leave the tube with its cuff beyond the anastomosis.

The above technique works well for lesions of the upper trachea. It is less satisfactory when the stricture or tumour is low in the trachea because the distal segment is so short that direct intubation locates the endotracheal tube in one or other of the main bronchi. A one-lung anaesthetic is entirely satisfactory for the brief period required to complete the tracheal suture line, provided the tube inserted through the wound is correctly situated and does not obstruct a lobar bronchus on the intubated side. The proximity of the right upper lobe orifice to the carina means that left endobronchial intubation is preferred if it is technically feasible. Also if any unilateral intubation is necessary, particular care should be taken to suck out blood and debris on the opposite side before restoring ventilation to both lungs.

Jet or Venturi ventilation. The catheter is passed into the airway either through the endotracheal tube from the proximal end, or is threaded directly into the airway, beyond the stenosis, by the surgeon. The endotracheal tube can then be partially withdrawn, away from the surgical field, and the tip of the catheter is secured with a stay-stitch in the distal tracheal segment to prevent it slipping into a main bronchus. If this does occur, ventilation will be restricted to only one lung and, although this may be acceptable in terms of gas exchange, there is a danger of pneumothorax or air embolism if the catheter moves further into the bronchial tree and impacts in a segmental division.

Satisfactory gas exchange can be maintained via a simple hand-held Venturi device or a high frequency jet ventilator while the anastomosis is completed, and anaesthesia is continued with intravenous agents, given intermittently or by infusion. The catheter is withdrawn as soon as the tracheal anastomosis has been completed, and ventilation is continued through the endotracheal tube which is advanced sufficiently to ensure that its cuff lies below the cords.

Resection of tumours at the carina poses particular problems. It is usually possible to maintain the airway at first by endotracheal intubation but, in some instances, it is necessary to pass an endobronchial tube past the obstruction. This can only be done safely under direct vision because of the distortion which is likely to be present and the risk of haemorrhage if the tumour is damaged. Ventilation is managed during the resection either by separate intubation of both main bronchi or by jet ventilation. If the former is chosen, separate endotracheal tubes are inserted directly into each transected main bronchus and are joined to the anaesthetic circuit with a double-lumen connector. It is difficult to avoid occluding the right upper lobe with this arrangement and it may be preferable to accept unilateral ventilation to the left lung. This will be necessary in any case while the right main bronchus is sutured to the lower end of the remaining trachea. Once this has been completed, the original endotracheal tube can be advanced just beyond the anastomosis and ventilation continued to the right lung while the left main bronchus is sutured to the trachea higher up.

One-lung anaesthesia results in a considerable shunt of desaturated blood through the unventilated side and, if there is any real anxiety about gas exchange during left lung anaesthesia, it may be preferable to consider a jet ventilation technique. Both lungs can be ventilated for longer periods if jet ventilation is chosen because two catheters, each placed separately in a main bronchus, occupy very little space. There is, however, a greater chance of contaminating the distal bronchial tree with blood.

Postoperative care

There are conflicting requirements in the postoperative period and it can be difficult to decide which takes priority. Bronchial secretions must be cleared efficiently to prevent atelectasis and infection which might progress to respiratory failure and hence require mechanical ventilation. This is regarded as particularly undesirable because positive pressure could weaken the recently completed suture line; HFJV is a theoretically attractive alternative. Tracheostomy and long-term endotracheal intubation are obviously undesirable following tracheal resection but if clearance of secretions is likely to be a problem a mini-tracheotomy tube can be placed through the cricothyroid membrane at the end of surgery.

These factors should be discussed for each patient individually, making allowance at the same time for other variables such as hypersecretion of mucus in those with a proven history of generalized airway disease, difficulty with expectoration if one recurrent laryngeal nerve has been sacrificed, and defective clearance mechanisms if the mucociliary blanket has been destroyed because of a need to bridge a long gap in the trachea with a plastic prosthesis. In general, every attempt should be made to restore efficient spontaneous ventilation, to extubate the patient straight away, and to achieve adequate pain relief and good humidification so that the patient can keep his own respiratory tract free from secretions. A stout suture is often used to keep the head flexed and so avoid unnecessary tension on the tracheal suture line.

INTRATRACHEAL STENTS

Intratracheal, or respiratory, stents are used to keep compromised large airways open in a variety of malignant and benign conditions. Malignant tumours can cause airway narrowing by either extrinsic compression or direct invasion and both these situations may be palliated by the insertion of intratracheal stents. Benign causes of airway obstruction amenable to stenting include anastomotic stricture (for example following sleeve resection or lung transplantation), postirradiation damage, tracheobronchial malacia, postintubation stricture and traumatic injury. A variety of different stents are available, the most commonly used being made of a suitable size of silicone rubber tubing with or without a T-piece extension to protrude through a tracheostomy. More recently, expandable metal stents, made from a mesh of stainless steel wire, have been introduced.

The anaesthetic considerations for the insertion and positioning of intratracheal stents are similar to those described for laser bronchoscopy (see Chapter 3) as difficulties with ventilation and maintenance of the airway are of most concern. Anaesthesia is maintained intravenously with a continuous infusion of propofol and paralysis is provided initially with suxamethonium followed by atracurium or vecuronium once the airway has been secured bronchoscopically. An inhalational induction may be used, but is rarely necessary. Maintenance of anaesthesia breathing spontaneously is imprac-tical for this type of procedure.

The stents are positioned using a rigid bronchoscope and Venturi ventilation can be employed in most situations, although HFJV is a possible alternative. It is essential to ensure that expiration can occur whichever mode of ventilation is used otherwise barotrauma will ensue with disastrous consequences. Wire metal stents are compressed in an introducing catheter, which can be passed down a rigid bronchoscope, but bulkier silicone rubber stents may need to be introduced directly through the larynx with the aid of a laryngoscope and forceps. Once through the larynx these latter stents are advanced and positioned with grasping forceps placed through the distal end of a bronchoscope. The airway may be totally blocked at times and cooperation is required between the anaesthetist and surgeon to ensure that significant hypoxia does not occur. It will be necessary to remove the stent and reventilate the patient in some instances and it may take several attempts before the stent is optimally positioned. In extreme circumstances partial, femoral vein to femoral artery, cardiopulmonary bypass has been used to augment oxygenation prior to insertion of an intratracheal stent.

A T-tube (Montgomery) is used to stent strictures of the cervical trachea. The T-portion of the tube protrudes through the neck via a tracheostomy, providing a site for suction and also serving to anchor the stent in place. The patient is initially anaesthetized via an endotracheal tube whilst the trache-ostomy is fashioned. The endotracheal tube is then removed and the distal and proximal limbs of the T-tube are introduced through the tracheostomy with forceps. The T-limb is pulled through the tracheostomy and final placement of the tube is carried out via a rigid bronchoscope placed through the larynx. Once the distal limb is open it is possible to utilize Venturi ventilation via the open limb of the T-tube. This site can also be used for ventilation in those patients returning for a change of T-tube.

Once a stent is in place anaesthesia is discontinued and the patient allowed to breathe spontaneously in a sitting position. Airway patency should be improved by the procedure but there may be short-term problems relating to the presence of blood and secretions in addition to general airway trauma. Respiratory stents can move and this may lead to acute airway obstruction which requires immediate re-operation.

REPAIR OF RUPTURED AIRWAYS

It is unusual for the trachea or main bronchi to be ruptured in isolation, although the larynx and upper trachea are vulnerable to knife and gunshot wounds. Damage to the lower trachea or the major bronchi is often associated with injuries to the chest wall, diaphragm, and thoracic viscera which influence overall management to such an extent that the principles outlined below need modification.

Injuries to the larynx and trachea

Control of the airway is the chief requirement, both at the time of presentation and during preparation for surgery. Endotracheal intubation is best attempted under local anaesthesia with the patient awake, or using spontaneous respiration with an oxygen and halothane mixture. The nature and location of the injury can be determined and the feasibility of intubation assessed without compromising the airway or using positive pressure. If intubation proves impossible and the lesion is high in the trachea or larynx, tracheostomy can be attempted under local anaesthesia. Alternatively the airway can be explored under direct vision with a bronchoscope.

Bronchial rupture

This rare injury usually occurs just above or below the carina, often as a result of chest compression. There is almost always mediastinal and surgical emphysema, pneumothorax and haemopneumothorax are common, and pneumopericardium with tamponade occurs occasionally. A pneumothorax which persists after trauma, in spite of a large chest drain through which there is a considerable air leak, is very suggestive of bronchial rupture and full expansion of a lung does not exclude the possibility of bronchial transection. Many cases present less acutely, and bronchial rupture is often diagnosed a considerable time after the injury when bronchoscopy is undertaken to investigate a persistently collapsed lobe or lung. Bronchial repair in these circumstances presents few hazards because endobronchial intubation of the opposite side provides control of the airway, but it may prove impossible to salvage the lobe or lung if longstanding obstruction has led to irreversible changes.

Management of those presenting acutely at the time of injury is much more difficult. Endotracheal intubation is often carried out as an emergency because of respiratory distress in a patient with multiple injuries. IPPV should be avoided if at all possible before any pneumothoraces have been drained but, even after a chest drain has been inserted, a large air leak from the ruptured bronchus can still interfere with ventilation to the uninjured lung and the pneumothorax can still develop tension if the air leak is large relative to the size of the drain. It is preferable, but not always practical, to retain spontaneous respiration until the site of rupture has been isolated by passing an endobronchial tube beyond it into the opposite lung. This is bound to be difficult, even under direct vision in an adult, and it may be preferable to maintain gentle IPPV by hand through an endotracheal tube while urgent preparations are made for immediate thoracotomy so that the site of the air leak can be controlled. Endobronchial intubation is possible in children but can only be undertaken blindly and so is even less satisfactory.

It is usually easy to ventilate the lungs as soon as the rupture has been repaired, but the presence of other injuries may necessitate mechanical ventilation postoperatively. This probably carries few risks because the recently completed suture line is supported by the re-expanded lung, and the pleural cavity will remain drained until any air leaks are sealed.

TRACHEO-OESOPHAGEAL FISTULA IN THE ADULT

Tracheo-oesophageal fistula is seen occasionally in adult patients as a consequence of trauma, neoplasm, or prolonged intubation. These patients are often seriously ill and pneumonia and even lung abscess are common. The principles governing their management are straightforward and it is usually possible to isolate the fistula at the time of induction with either a long endotracheal tube or a double-lumen endobronchial tube. Congenital tracheo-oesophageal fistula commonly presents in the neonatal period and the reader is referred to specialized paediatric texts for a description of the management of this condition.

OESOPHAGEAL SURGERY

The oesophagus is a muscular tube which runs from the pharynx to the stomach. There is an upper oesophageal sphincter which closes off the pharynx from the upper oesophagus by way of the cricopharyngeus muscle and also a lower oesophageal sphincter (LOS) which has important anaesthetic implications. The LOS is the major barrier preventing reflux from the stomach into the lower oesophagus. Other mechanisms preventing regurgitation include the valve effect created by the angle at which the oesophagus joins the stomach and the closure or 'pinch-cock' effect exerted by the right crus of the diaphragm.

The LOS is an area of circular muscle fibres 2–5 cm in length innervated via the parasympathetic system. In normal subjects the LOS extends above and below the diaphragm and its pressure increases in response to an elevation of intra-abdominal pressure, thereby maintaining a constant barrier pressure between the stomach and oesophagus. Patients with oesophageal disease may have abnormalities of LOS function so that regurgitation of stomach contents is more likely, particularly at induction of anaesthesia. In addition, drug therapy (Table 9.1) and a number of hormones are known to affect LOS tone and their effect should be taken into consideration in patients presenting for oesophageal investigation and surgery.

Prevention of aspiration at induction of anaesthesia for oesophageal

Table 9.1 Effects of drugs on lower oesophageal sphincter tone. From Aitkenhead (1987)

Increase	Decrease	No change
Metoclopramide	Atropine	Propranolol
Domperidone	Glycopyrrolate	Oxprenolol
Prochlorperazine	Dopamine	Cimetidine
Cyclizine	Sodium nitroprusside	Ranitidine
Edrophonium	Ganglion blockers	Atracurium
Neostigmine	Thiopentone	? Nitrous oxide
Histamine	Tricyclic antidepressants	
Suxamethonium	β-Adrenergic agonists	
Pancuronium	Halothane	
Metoprolol	Enflurane	
α-Adrenergic agonists	Opioids	
Antacids	? Nitrous oxide	

surgery is predominantly by means of a rapid sequence induction, with cricoid pressure applied to occlude the oesophageal lumen. Alternatively, the head-up position is advocated by some anaesthetists to prevent regurgitation in patients with a hiatus hernia. In patients with a large dilated oesophagus containing food debris it may be safer to empty the oesophagus via the rigid oesophagoscope a few days before elective surgery. This latter procedure also carries a risk, however.

Antacids may be given to increase gastric pH but drugs such as magnesium trisilicate are white and viscous and therefore are likely to obscure the surgeon's view if oesophagoscopy is planned. Sodium citrate (30 ml of a 0.3 molar solution given 30 minutes prior to surgery) avoids this problem but should be administered in combination with H_2 receptor antagonists, given orally the night before and on the day of surgery, to ascertain that gastric pH is sufficiently raised to prevent an acid-aspiration syndrome. The role of proton pump inhibitors such as omeprazole in lowering gastric acid secretion in the acute preoperative situation has yet to be defined, but they should be continued up to the time of surgery if patients are taking them chronically. Oral metoclopramide may also facilitate gastric emptying whilst maintaining LOS pressure (Table 9.1).

Repair of hiatus hernia

This common condition is asymptomatic in up to 50% of cases and the majority of symptomatic patients are treated medically. Surgery is needed in a small proportion, the usual indications being failed medical treatment, dysphagia because a stricture has formed, haemorrhage, or recurrent aspiration into the respiratory tract (Fig. 9.5). Several operations have been described, all intended to produce a valvular effect at the oesophagogastric junction; dilatation of a stricture may be needed at the same time. Emergency surgery is required occasionally in patients with a rolling-type hiatus hernia which incarcerates and strangulates within the chest. These patients present with acute chest pain and vomiting and are often shocked and dehydrated on admission. Hydration and electrolyte disturbances should be corrected before operation and antibiotic treatment initiated to prevent the development of mediastinitis.

Patients with a hiatus hernia presenting for elective repair should be operated on when they have achieved an optimum weight. Correction of obesity is necessary more often than nutritional supplements. Antacids are continued preoperatively but white, viscous preparations are substituted with sodium citrate (see above) so that the oesophageal mucosa is not obscured if

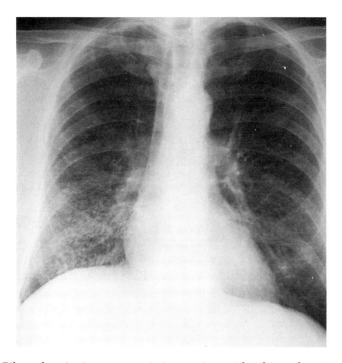

Fig. 9.5 Bilateral aspiration pneumonia in a patient with a hiatus hernia and oesophageal stricture.

preoperative oesophagoscopy is required. Oral or intravenous H_2 antagonists can be given on the evening prior to surgery and at the time of premedication to raise the pH of the gastric contents.

Anaesthesia for repair of hiatus hernia

Precautions should be taken at the time of induction to prevent regurgitation and aspiration of gastric contents. If this risk is regarded as small, it is reasonable to use a double-lumen endobronchial tube, rather than an endotracheal tube, so that one-lung ventilation can be used if necessary. The operation is carried out through a left thoracotomy but a left-sided, double-lumen tube is entirely satisfactory and carries little risk of obstructing a lobar bronchus. An endotracheal rather than an endobronchial tube should be chosen if intubation must be carried out quickly because the risks of regurgitation and aspiration are high, for example, in patients with an incarcerated hernia. A double-lumen tube will be inconvenient if oesophagoscopy precedes the thoracotomy because it occupies too much space.

However, there is usually little difficulty if the sole requirement is to pass a bougie or large nasogastric tube through the hernia or stricture so that the oesophagus is easier to mobilize and manipulate.

The general principles of anaesthesia during thoracotomy (Chapters 4 and 5) apply during oesophageal surgery. It is important to note, however, that statistically hypoxaemia is more likely to be severe and protracted if the left lung is collapsed throughout oesophageal surgery than when lung resection is undertaken. Insufflation of oxygen to the unventilated lung, at a pressure of approximately $5–10\,cmH_2O$, lessens the severity of hypoxaemia without compromising surgical access (see Fig. 4.4). However, oesophageal surgery of this type can be carried out while both lungs are ventilated, and the degree of retraction of the left lung necessary for adequate access causes less reduction in the arterial oxygen tension than one-lung anaesthesia.

Blood loss is rarely heavy but the repair entails extensive dissection and mobilization of the oesophagus and proximal stomach. Disturbances of cardiac rhythm and hiccup are more common than during operations on the lung, but both usually respond to simple measures. It is usually possible to re-establish spontaneous ventilation at the end of the operation but adequate pain relief is particularly important postoperatively because the intra-abdominal disturbance may cause distension which interferes with re-expansion of the left lung.

Achalasia of the cardia

This is a generalized disorder of oesophageal motility characterized by incoordinate or absent peristalsis. The tone of the LOS is normal or slightly elevated, and the dilated oesophagus, full of secretions and food residues, is often ulcerated (Fig. 9.6). Repeated episodes of aspiration into the lungs occur, often at night, causing 'asthma', bronchopneumonia and lung abscess.

Heller's operation, or oesophageal myotomy, is the preferred surgical treatment and involves incision of the circular muscle of the cardia and lower end of the oesophagus. Reflux may be induced as a result and may need to be controlled by an additional anti-reflux procedure carried out at the same time. The chief hazard of anaesthesia is aspiration of the contents of the dilated oesophagus into the lungs, but this can be avoided by preoperative preparation (see text above and Fig. 9.7). A grossly dilated and abnormal oesophagus such as those shown in Figs 9.6 and 9.7 may require excision and replacement with either stomach or colon. This is obviously much more extensive surgery than a myotomy and anaesthesia is conducted on the lines described below for oesophagectomy.

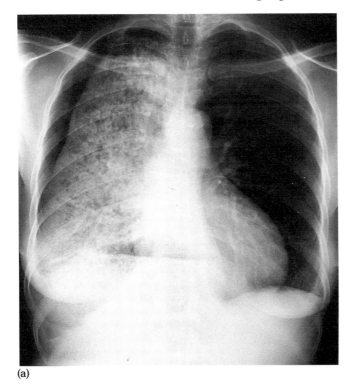

(a)

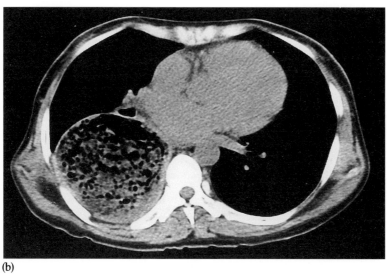

(b)

Fig. 9.6 (a) Chest X-ray of a female patient with achalasia of the oesophagus. (b) CT scan of the same patient. The grossly dilated oesophagus fills a large proportion of the right chest and is full of food debris.

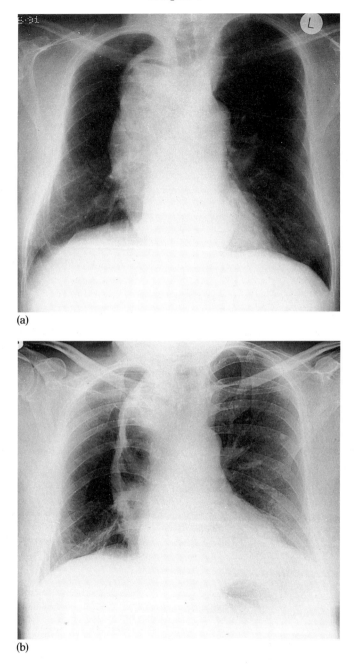

(a)

(b)

Fig. 9.7 Chest X-rays of a male patient with achalasia (a) before and (b) after food debris has been cleared at oesophagoscopy.

Carcinoma of the oesophagus

Severe, progressive dysphagia is the characteristic symptom of oesophageal carcinoma at any level. A high proportion of patients have irresectable disease at the time of presentation and palliative treatment is all that can be offered. Insertion of an oesophageal tube, either at laparotomy or by pulsion intubation of the oesophagus at endoscopy, provides some temporary relief but the quality of palliation is poor and the mortality of the procedure high. Operation to bypass the tumour is gaining in popularity: the stomach is mobilized through a midline abdominal incision and, after division and closure of the cardia, is passed behind the sternum into the neck. The oesophagus is transected and closed above the tumour and the fundus of the stomach is anastomosed to the pharynx or proximal oesophagus in the neck. The incidence of complication is far lower than after oesophageal resection, the quality of palliation is superior and, because the stomach is well away from the diseased oesophagus, there are fewer constraints on the dose of irradiation if control of the growth is to be attempted.

Carcinoma of the lower or middle third of the oesophagus can be treated by resection in a proportion of patients but it is a major procedure, usually carried out through a left thoraco-abdominal incision. Stomach, jejunum or colon are used to restore the continuity of the alimentary tract, but the immediate mortality of all current procedures is high — of the order of 10–20%. Endoscopic oesophageal resection is still in the development phase and not yet an established technique.

Good preoperative preparation is essential before surgery of this magnitude. Starvation and nutritional oedema progress to dehydration when even liquids, including saliva, cannot be swallowed, and chronic haemorrhage adds to the anaemia and hypoproteinaemia. These weak, debilitated, and often elderly patients are prone to infection, their wounds heal poorly and anastomotic leaks are common. Every effort should be made to improve nutrition preoperatively, using a liquid diet if the stricture permits or a parenteral regime. The latter should be continued postoperatively until oral feeding is resumed.

Anaesthesia for oesophagectomy

There are few constraints on premedication or the choice of anaesthetic agents, provided allowance is made for age and nutritional status. A double-lumen left-sided endobronchial tube during operation allows deflation of the left lung when necessary and during a long procedure it may be prudent to insufflate oxygen to this lung.

Blood and fluid loss can be considerable during oesophagectomy and a multiple-lumen central venous catheter is mandatory to provide a reliable route for both drug and fluid therapy in addition to the measurement of venous pressure. Any existing line which has been inserted for parenteral feeding should be reserved solely for this purpose and one side of the neck should be left entirely free in case surgical access is required to create the upper anastomosis. In many cases it is sensible to insert central venous catheters in the femoral vein well away from the site of surgery. A wide-bore venous cannula should also be inserted to provide a route for rapid transfusion. Full monitoring should be instituted as for any major thoracic surgery (see Chapter 5). This will include as a minimum an ECG, pulse oximetry, an indwelling arterial line with continuous display of blood pressure and measurement of central venous pressure, urine output and central temperature.

The operation is often prolonged and difficult and the thoraco-abdominal incision provides a large surface for heat loss. All transfused fluids should be warmed, inspired gases warmed and humidified, and body temperature monitored throughout. Crystalloids should only be given cautiously because hypoproteinaemic patients often have an increase in total body water and tolerate fluid overload very poorly. A nasogastric tube should be available towards the end of the operation so that it can be threaded through the anastomosis and into the stomach if the surgeon wishes. Its purpose is to prevent gastric distension and indicate if bleeding is continuing from the stomach; it provides no guarantee against aspiration of gastric contents into the lungs. The tube is uncomfortable and interferes with coughing so some surgeons prefer to use a pharyngogastric tube or leave the stomach undrained.

Fit patients can be allowed to breathe spontaneously after an uncomplicated procedure, but these cases are in a minority. Patients should not be extubated until alert and sitting upright, as there is no mechanical barrier to reflux and aspiration into the lungs is a major hazard postoperatively. Epidural analgesia will help a spontaneously breathing patient to maintain satisfactory, pain-free, ventilation. Debilitated, elderly subjects in particular benefit if mechanical ventilation is continued for 12–24 hours, especially after a long operation. Sedation can be used to control pain without fear of respiratory depression, efficient bronchial toilet can be carried out, and spontaneous ventilation can be re-established in optimum circumstances the next day when blood volume, fluid balance, renal function, and acid–base status have all been corrected as far as possible. In this latter group of patients it is still useful to insert an epidural catheter at the time of surgery to provide pain relief during the periods of mechanical ventilation and the weaning process.

FURTHER READING

Removal of foreign bodies

Baraka A. (1974) Bronchoscopic removal of foreign bodies in children. *British Journal of Anaesthesia,* **46** 124–126.

Bready L.L., Orr M.D., Petty C., Grover F.L. & Harman K. (1986) Bronchoscopic administration of racemic adrenaline to facilitate removal of aspired peanut fragments in pediatric patients. *Anesthesiology,* **65,** 523–525.

Griffiths D.M. & Freeman N.V. (1984) Expiratory chest X-ray examination in the diagnosis of inhaled foreign bodies. *British Medical Journal,* **288,** 1074–1075.

Lloyd-Thomas J.A. & Bush G.H. (1986) All that wheezes is not asthma. *Anaesthesia,* **41,** 181–185.

Maharaj R.J., Whitton I. & Blyth D. (1983) Emergency extracorporeal oxygenation for an intratracheal foreign body. *Anaesthesia,* **38,** 471–474.

Mearns A.J. & England R.M. (1975) Dissolving foreign bodies in the trachea and bronchus, *Thorax,* **30,** 461–463.

Sloan I.A. & Alberti, P.W. (1982) Foreign bodies in the respiratory tract of children. *Annals of the Royal College of Surgeons of England,* **64,** 201–204.

Tracheal stenosis and tracheal resection

El-Baz N., Holinger L., El-Ganzouri A., Gottschalk W. & Ivankovich A.D. (1982) High-frequency positive pressure ventilation for tracheal reconstruction supported by tracheal T-tube. *Anesthesia and Analgesia,* **61,** 796–800.

Murphy P.N. & Lloyd-Thomas A. (1991) The anaesthetic management of congenital tracheal stenosis. *Anaesthesia,* **46,** 106–109.

Rogers R.C., Gibbons J., Cosgrove J. & Coppel D.L. (1985) High-frequency jet ventilation for tracheal surgery. *Anaesthesia,* **40,** 32–36.

Smith G.A., Castresana M.R. & Mandel S.D. (1983) Ventilatory management of tracheomalacia utilising high-frequency jet ventilation. *Anesthesia and Analgesia,* **62,** 538–540.

Wilson R.F., Steiger Z., Jacobs J., Sison O.S. & Holsey C. (1984) Temporary partial cardiopulmonary bypass during emergency operative management of near total tracheal occlusion. *Anesthesiology,* **61,** 103–105.

Young-Beyer P. & Wilson R.S. (1988) Anesthetic management for tracheal resection and reconstruction. *Journal of Cardiothoracic Anesthesia,* **2,** 821–835.

Intratracheal stents

George P.J.M. & Rudd R.M. (1992) Respiratory stents. *British Journal of Hospital Medicine,* **47,** 426–429.

Sherry K.M., Keeling P.A., Jones H.M. & Aveling W. (1987) Insertion of intratracheal stents. Anaesthetic management using high-frequency jet ventilation or cardiopulmonary bypass. *Anaesthesia,* **42,** 61–66.

Unger M. (1990) Tracheobronchial stents and shunts. *Chest,* **97,** 260–261.

Repair of ruptured airways

Alfille P.H. & Hurford W.E. (1991) Upper airway injuries. *Journal of Clinical Anesthesia*, **3**, 88–90.
Bertelsen S. & Howitz P. (1972) Injuries of the trachea and bronchi. *Thorax*, **27**, 188–194.
Cicala R.S., Kudsk K.A., Butts A., Nguyen H. & Fabian T. (1991) Initial evaluation and management of upper airway injuries in trauma patients. *Journal of Clinical Anesthesia*, **3**, 91–97.
Mathisen D.J. & Grillo H. (1987) Laryngotracheal trauma. *Annals of Thoracic Surgery*, **43**, 254–262.

Oesophageal surgery

Aitkenhead A.R. (1987) Anaesthesia for oesophageal surgery. In: Gothard J.W.W. (ed.) *Thoracic Anaesthesia. Clinical Anaesthesiology*, Vol. 1, pp. 181–206. Baillière Tindall, London.
Dickerson J.W.T. (1984) Nutrition in the cancer patient: a review. *Journal of the Royal Society of Medicine*, **77**, 309–315.
Evans J.M., Davies W.L. & Wise C.C. (1984) Lower oesophageal contractility: a new monitor of anaesthesia. *Lancet*, **i**, 1151–1154.
Gothard J.W.W. (1993) Thoracic surgery. In: Aitkenhead A.R. & Jones R.M. (eds) *Anaesthesia in Clinical Practice*. Churchill Livingstone, Edinburgh.
Grebenik C.R. (1989) Anaesthetic management of malignant tracheo-oesophageal fistula. *British Journal of Anaesthesia*, **63**, 492–496.
Orringer M.B. (1989) Ten-year survival after esophagectomy for carcinoma. Surgical triumph or biologic variation? *Chest*, **96**, 970–971.
Travis K.W., Saini V.K. & O'Sullivan P.T. (1981) Upper airway obstruction and achalasia of the esophagus. *Anesthesiology*, **54**, 87–88.

10: Miscellaneous Procedures

BRONCHOPULMONARY LAVAGE

This term is used in a number of circumstances to describe the instillation and subsequent removal of a solution (usually normal saline) into the bronchial tree. Aliquots of 25–50 ml are used to retrieve cells from the alveoli during fibreoptic bronchoscopy and similar quantities can be instilled and aspirated repeatedly to remove mucous plugs in patients with severe asthma. The term is used here to describe the use of many litres of saline to eliminate unwanted material from the alveolar spaces.

The usual indication for this treatment is alveolar proteinosis (Fig. 10.1), a rare disease in which lipoprotein accumulates within the lung without provoking any sort of inflammatory or fibrotic response within the alveolar walls. Inhaled, insoluble radioactive substances can also be removed in this way if treatment is instituted soon enough after the accident, but lavage is no longer used to remove the inspissated sputum of patients with bronchiectasis or cystic fibrosis because it is often followed by fever and hypotension.

Progressive dyspnoea, an unproductive cough and malaise are the usual symptoms of alveolar proteinosis and, although spontaneous remission does occur, most patients deteriorate relentlessly. The diagnosis is often established late when severe hypoxaemia and secondary polycythaemia are already present; most patients also receive corticosteroids because the condition is confused with sarcoidosis or pulmonary fibrosis. However,

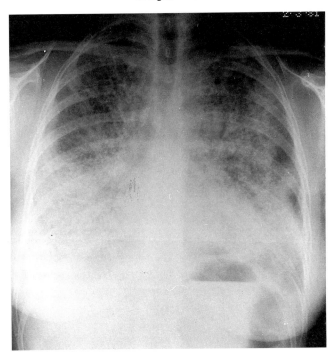

Fig. 10.1 Alveolar proteinosis in a woman of 43. Gas transfer was reduced to approximately 25% of predicted and the arterial oxygen tension, breathing air, was 3.8 kPa. Successful bronchopulmonary lavage was undertaken, using 40 litres of saline on each side.

hypoxaemia develops gradually and so there is time for compensatory mechanisms to develop too. The metabolic rate is not elevated, as it might be when a comparable degree of hypoxaemia occurs as a result of infection or trauma; thus the hazards of one-lung anaesthesia are less than might be anticipated.

Anaesthetic management and technique of lavage

The two sides are treated on separate occasions, usually 1 week apart. Anaesthesia and ventilation are maintained through one lung while the other side is treated. Isolation of the two lungs must be perfect and this can be achieved most reliably if a left-sided, double-lumen tube is always used, whichever side is being treated. In exceptional circumstances (e.g. if lavage is required in a child too small for intubation with a double-lumen tube) the procedure can be carried out during cardiopulmonary bypass. Cardiopulmonary bypass can usually be avoided in children, however, by placing a Foley catheter in the lavage lung whilst ventilation is maintained to the contralateral lung via a rigid bronchoscope within the trachea. A relatively effective washout can then be achieved via the Foley catheter.

The patient should be premedicated cautiously, especially if severely hypoxaemic. Preoxygenation is followed by an intravenous induction, and a non-depolarizing muscle relaxant (e.g. vecuronium) is given to provide good conditions for endobronchial intubation and a smooth transition to controlled ventilation. 100% oxygen is used throughout, not only to ensure adequate oxygenation while ventilation is being maintained through a single poorly functioning lung, but also to promote complete uptake of gas within the treated lung. Isoflurane is a suitable maintenance agent.

The patient lies supine with the treated side slightly dependent — a posture which decreases the chance of saline entering the ventilated lung and also limits gravitational redistribution of pulmonary blood flow to the unventilated lung (Fig. 10.2). Some centres place the patient in a Stryker frame to allow rotation of the patient and a more efficient washout. The side to be treated is excluded from the anaesthetic circuit at the end of an

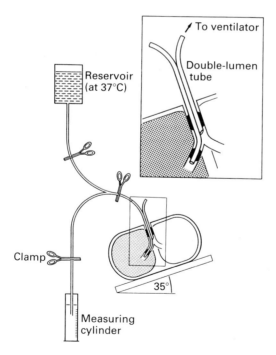

Fig. 10.2 Diagram illustrating the circuit used for bronchopulmonary lavage.

expiration; normal saline, buffered to a pH of 7.4 and warmed to approximately body temperature, is allowed to run into the lung at 1 minute intervals from a reservoir approximately 45 cm above the table, delivering a volume each minute equal to the anticipated oxygen uptake through that lung. This is continued until the treated lung has been filled with a volume of saline equal to its functional residual capacity, calculated as 55 or 45% respectively for the right and left lungs of the total functional residual capacity measured preoperatively. Increments of saline of between 500 and 1000 ml are run in and out thereafter until the fluid returning is clear. Between 20 and 40 litres are necessary in most cases to produce a clear effluent. Serial measurements of protein concentration in this effluent may indicate, however, that a clinically satisfactory endpoint has been reached well before 40 litres of wash have been used. At the end of the procedure, residual saline is drained from the lung, ventilation is restored to both sides and mechanical ventilation is continued for a few hours while the saline left inside the lung (usually no more than 200–300 ml) is absorbed.

Disturbances to the blood volume and its electrolyte composition do not occur but it is essential to monitor oxygen saturation and end-tidal carbon dioxide levels throughout the procedure, in addition to the electrocardiogram and non-invasive blood pressure measurements. The arterial oxygen tension during one-lung anaesthesia with isoflurane in 100% oxygen and the opposite lung filled with saline is at least equal to and usually greater than the preoperative value while breathing air. It is rarely necessary to require invasive arterial monitoring or a pulmonary artery catheter. The greatest risk of significant hypoxaemia is during re-expansion of the treated lung, when pulmonary blood flow increases on that side after being partially obstructed during treatment by the hydrostatic pressure of the lavage fluid. Serious hypoxaemia is most unlikely during the lavage; if it does occur, the probable cause is either that the endobronchial portion of the double-lumen tube is obstructing a lobar bronchus on the intubated side or that saline has penetrated the intubated lung. Both can be avoided by meticulous attention to detail. Repeated lavage may be necessary at intervals over many years but, in spite of the obvious hazards, the results are excellent and the anaesthetist has the privilege of restoring a disabled patient to normal health.

MEDIASTINAL TUMOURS

Mediastinal tumours are rare but tend to present to specialized thoracic centres for diagnostic biopsy or resection (see Mediastinoscopy — Chapter 3). The commonest tumours are neural in origin (Figs 10.3 and 10.4) followed in order by teratomata and thymic neoplasms. A number of other tumours

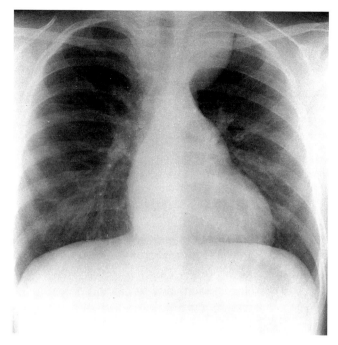

Fig. 10.3 Chest X-ray of a 6-year-old child presenting with a persistent cough. An opacity, which proved to be a ganglioneuroma, is seen at the apex of the left lung.

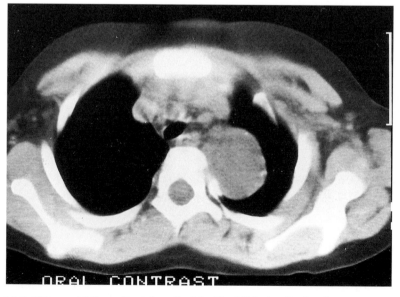

ORAL CONTRAST

Fig. 10.4 CT scan of the patient described in Fig. 10.3 clearly showing a mass adjacent to a vertebral body in the upper thorax.

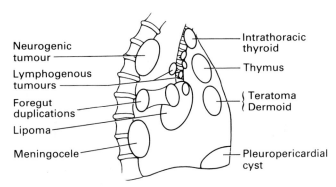

Neurogenic tumour

Lymphogenous tumours

Foregut duplications

Lipoma

Meningocele

Intrathoracic thyroid

Thymus

Teratoma
Dermoid

Pleuropericardial cyst

Fig. 10.5 Sites of mediastinal tumours (Gothard, 1989).

occurring in the mediastinum include lymphomata, pleuropericardial cysts and intrathoracic goitre (Fig. 10.5).

Mediastinal tumours, particularly those in the anterior mediastinum, may cause a variety of difficulties during anaesthesia which are described below. Anaesthesia for thymectomy in patients with myasthenia gravis is discussed separately.

Anaesthesia for biopsy and resection of anterior mediastinal tumours

Major anaesthetic problems encountered with anterior mediastinal tumours include airway obstruction, compression of intrathoracic vascular structures and the effects of preoperative radiotherapy and chemotherapy. Intraoperative bleeding may also be severe and adequate central intravenous access should be established in both the superior vena cava (SVC) and inferior vena cava (IVC), in case the former system is damaged or clamped during surgery.

Airway obstruction

Tumour compression of the trachea and main bronchi causes airway obstruction. Patients with an anterior mediastinal tumour commonly present with a cough, dyspnoea and difficulty in breathing, particularly when lying flat. Tracheal compression may be evident on the chest X-ray (Fig. 10.6) and this can be further evaluated by CT (Fig. 10.7) and magnetic resonance scanning. Pulmonary function tests will confirm airway obstruction.

North American authors have advocated the use of preoperative radiotherapy or chemotherapy in those patients with severe upper airway

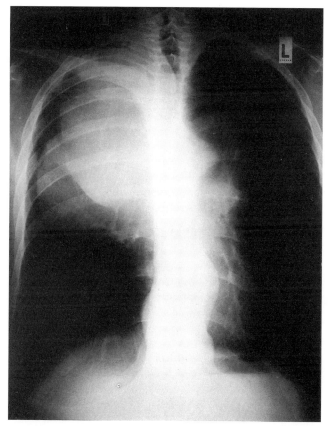

Fig. 10.6 Chest X-ray of a male patient with a large mediastinal tumour. Obvious tracheal narrowing is present.

obstruction, given, if necessary, without a firm histological diagnosis. This has not been accepted practice in the UK where every effort is made to establish a tissue diagnosis before treatment, which may mask pathological characteristics of the tumour, is started. There is a risk of severe and even fatal intraoperative respiratory obstruction but this can be minimized by careful planning. This risk is considered justifiable in the context of patients with extremely aggressive tumours whose long-term treatment and survival depend on an accurate histological diagnosis. Ferrari and Bedford, 1990, (Sloan–Kettering Cancer Center, New York) have recently expressed similar views and reported their experience in 44 children with anterior mediastinal tumours.

Classically, it is taught that anaesthesia should be induced inhalationally in the presence of upper airway obstruction. This approach creates a number

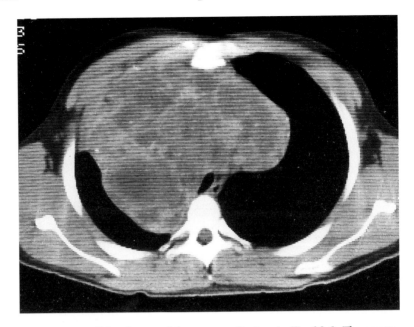

Fig. 10.7 CT scan of the thorax of the same patient as in Fig. 10.6. The narrow trachea is seen posterior to a large mass.

of problems if the obstruction is due to extrinsic compression by an anterior mediastinal mass. Lung volume is reduced during anaesthesia and bronchial smooth muscle relaxes, thereby increasing the compressibility of the large airways. Partially obstructed respiration, which is not uncommon during an inhalational induction, generates large negative intrathoracic pressures which will further tend to flatten an airway weakened by extrinsic compression. In the majority of patients an intravenous induction can be carried out in the sitting position, following preoxygenation. After muscle relaxation with suxamethonium a rigid bronchoscope is passed through the externally compressed trachea and Venturi ventilation commenced. If compression of the airway is limited to the upper trachea an endotracheal tube can usually be passed through the stricture. Narrowing of the lower trachea or main bronchi may require the use of a longer armoured endotracheal tube, or even an endobronchial tube (single- or double-lumen), to negotiate the compression and allow ventilation. These latter tubes can be placed under direct vision using the fibreoptic or rigid intubating bronchoscope.

Femoral vein to femoral artery cardiopulmonary bypass, established under local anaesthesia, can be used to provide gas exchange during the resection of mediastinal tumours in those patients with severe airway obstruction. The main drawback to this technique is the increased risk of bleeding as a result of heparinization.

Spontaneous respiration can usually be established following tumour resection, despite the presence of an airway weakened by chronic compression. A period of mechanical ventilation may be indicated for other reasons such as phrenic nerve section, massive blood loss and prolonged surgery. After biopsy of a mediastinal tumour spontaneous respiration may be compromised because of the effects of anaesthesia in patients with pre-existing respiratory obstruction. Once spontaneous respiration has been satisfactorily established, with the patient in a sitting position, a trial of extubation can be carried out. A few patients will require emergency re-intubation followed by a period of mechanical ventilation. Removal of the endotracheal tube will be possible at a later stage in the majority of these patients once the effects of anaesthesia and surgery have receded. A very small number of patients will require treatment of their tumour either by radiotherapy, chemotherapy or surgery before they can be weaned from respiratory support. This latter group are in a very high-risk category but at least their treatment can be managed with the benefit of accurate histology.

Compression of intrathoracic vascular structures

Superior vena caval obstruction is a common presenting feature of anterior mediastinal tumours. Compression of the heart and pulmonary arteries occurs less frequently, but has been implicated in the deaths of several patients at induction of anaesthesia.

Pulmonary artery compression is likely if cyanosis is evident in the presence of satisfactory pulmonary function. This is particularly true if the cyanosis is more marked in the supine position or occurs during the straining of defecation. Cardiac compression presents with the cardiovascular abnormalities associated with pericardial tamponade and is treated on similar principles. Pulmonary artery compression may be alleviated if the patient is anaesthetized in the sitting position. Unfortunately pulmonary artery occlusion may be most marked on the side in which ventilation is the least compromised. In this situation one lung can easily be inflated during anaesthesia but the patient becomes progressively cyanosed because of poor, or absent, blood flow to that lung. Severe pulmonary artery compression may be one of the few indications to use cardiopulmonary bypass prior to the induction of anaesthesia.

Superior vena caval obstruction can present a number of difficulties during anaesthesia. These include a slow induction time if intravenous agents are administered via arm veins, respiratory obstruction and difficulty with endotracheal intubation in the presence of an oedematous mucosa in the upper airway. None of these factors are absolute contraindications to intravenous anaesthesia if the patient is managed in the sitting position and the airway is secured as described above.

Previous chemotherapy and radiotherapy

Pulmonary damage due to bleomycin therapy has the most significance in the anaesthetic management of patients with a mediastinal tumour. Bleomycin is used in the treatment of a number of tumours including primary and secondary teratomata, both of which occur in the mediastinum. Pulmonary damage occurs in up to 10% or more of patients treated. It is a dose-related phenomenon which is particularly likely to occur in the elderly, in those with poor lung function and following radiotherapy. Symptoms of pulmonary damage including shortness of breath, cough and fever follow a variable time course, but often develop over a period of weeks following treatment. Fine reticular shadows are initially seen on the chest X-ray, but at a later stage more widespread changes may be seen with linear infiltrates and patchy atelectasis.

There is evidence that high inspired oxygen concentrations used during and after anaesthesia potentiate the toxic effects of bleomycin on the lung. Inspired oxygen concentrations should therefore be kept to the minimum necessary to provide satisfactory arterial oxygenation as judged on pulse oximetry and intermittent blood gas analysis. Anaesthesia should be avoided in patients known to have acute bleomycin lung toxicity.

MYASTHENIA GRAVIS AND THE MYASTHENIC SYNDROME

Myasthenia gravis and thymectomy

The clinical features of myasthenia gravis (Table 10.1) have been recognized for over a century but the pathophysiology has only been clarified recently. It has been established that there is a reduction in the number of acetyl-choline receptors at the neuromuscular junction, and antibody against such receptors is present in the plasma of a high proportion of patients with the disease. An autoimmune basis has been confirmed and, although the role of the thymus is poorly understood, up to 75% of patients are improved by thymectomy and may even achieve complete remission. A thymoma is present sometimes and is an indication for thymectomy, but surgery is also

Table 10.1 Features of the myasthenic syndrome and myasthenia gravis

Myasthenic syndrome	Myasthenia gravis
Clinical features	
Occurs mainly in men of an elderly age group. There is weakness and fatigability of proximal limb muscles and tendon reflexes are reduced or absent. There is a temporary increase in strength (for a few seconds) of weakened muscles in response to exercise	More common in women. Mean age of onset 26 years. Initial symptoms of muscle weakness usually relate to the ocular, oro-pharyngeal and limb muscle groups
Electromyography	
Greatly reduced twitch on a single maximal stimulus. Transient further depression of the response with repetitive stimuli at rates of 1–10/s is observed with marked facilitation during stimulation at higher rates. There is marked facilitation of the response to stimuli for several seconds after voluntary contraction	Normal or slightly reduced response to single twitch stimulus. Reduced response to repeated stimuli at high and low frequencies. Rapid fade with tetanic stimulation
Response to muscle relaxants	
Sensitivity to both non-depolarizing and depolarizing drugs	Sensitive to non-depolarizing drugs Resistant to depolarizing drugs
Anticholinesterase therapy	
Poor response	Good response
Pathological features	
Small-cell carcinoma of the bronchus usually present	Thymoma present in 20–25% of patients

undertaken when the disease is inadequately controlled by other means. A substantial number of the thymus glands removed show evidence of hyperplasia and approximately 15% incorporate a thymoma. Symptomatic relief is provided with anticholinesterases, and immunosuppression therapy with corticosteroids and azathioprine may also be used. Plasmapheresis is useful in a proportion of severely ill patients.

Anaesthetic implications of thymectomy

Weakness of the respiratory muscles and an inability to cough or swallow effectively are the symptoms which are likely to interfere with management during and after operation. Treatment with anticholinesterases provokes salivation and hypersecretion from the respiratory tract, and patients with myasthenia gravis respond abnormally to a number of anaesthetic agents, particularly muscle relaxants.

Preoperative assessment includes measurement of forced vital capacity before and after a regular oral dose of pyridostigmine, and more detailed investigation of pulmonary function is necessary in patients who have coincidental lung disease. Particular attention should also be given to the presence or absence of bulbar symptoms. The dose and frequency of the anticholinesterase regime should be noted, as well as details of past or current use of corticosteroids. Intercurrent infection should be sought and treated vigorously before operation, especially in those using corticosteroids or recently treated by plasmapheresis.

Myasthenic patients are unduly sensitive to many forms of central nervous system depressants and so premedication should be light and combined with intramuscular atropine to prevent excessive salivation. Anticholinesterases are continued preoperatively but can be reduced by approximately 20% on hospitalization, firstly to take into account the sedentary period and secondly to prevent overdosage immediately postoperatively, when the need for anticholinesterases may be substantially reduced. The last dose of pyridostigmine before surgery can be omitted if respiratory muscle weakness is not a prominent feature symptomatically, and the measured vital capacity is at least 1 litre when a dose of the drug is due. If pyridostigmine is required an intramuscular injection of 1/30th the normal oral dose can be given.

Patients with myasthenia gravis are exceedingly sensitive to non-depolarizing muscle relaxants and resistant to depolarizing drugs. Endotracheal intubation and controlled ventilation can usually be established without difficulty using an inhalational agent alone, or supplemented by a small dose of an intravenous induction agent or a parenteral narcotic. As myasthenics are sensitive to non-depolarizing muscle relaxants anaesthetists have, generally, avoided their use. Atracurium, however, with its spontaneous degradation via the Hofmann elimination pathway, has been used successfully to provide muscle relaxation in myasthenics. Reduced dosage can be employed, if neuromuscular transmission monitoring is used, without the need for reversal. Avoiding reversal is advantageous in this group of patients because they may be sensitive to the effects of anticholinesterases in the postoperative period. Despite this, vecuronium has been used, in reduced dosage, to provide muscle relaxation for myasthenics and most reports cite the use of neostigmine for reversal.

Thymectomy for myasthenia can be undertaken via a transcervical/ suprasternal approach but some surgeons prefer a limited, upper, mediansternotomy. If the thymus is significantly enlarged a complete sternotomy may be necessary and this is certainly the correct approach if malignancy is suspected.

A period of postoperative mechanical ventilation is almost always necessary while residual anaesthetic agents are excreted and anticholinesterase therapy is re-established. Narcotic analgesics can be used to provide pain relief at reduced dosage during this period. Extubation is performed according to general principles, when the patient is awake and responsive and able to generate a negative pressure of −20 cm of water. A few patients, particularly those with severe disease and a previous history of respiratory failure, will require prolonged ventilation.

The return to spontaneous ventilation is usually smoother, and salivation and respiratory tract secretion less of a problem, if pyridostigmine can be given through a nasogastric tube in preference to atropine and neostigmine intravenously. Although there is usually no immediate reduction in the dose of anticholinesterase required, even a short period without the drug appears to enhance sensitivity and so care must be taken to avoid causing colic and hypersecretion, or even precipitating a cholinergic crisis. After extubation, physiotherapy should be timed to coincide with the maximum action of doses of anticholinesterase, with pain controlled using an inhalational agent such as Entonox. Regular physiotherapy is likely to be required for a number of days and particular vigilance is necessary to detect sputum retention early because many of these patients can never achieve a normal vital capacity and their treatment provokes an increase in secretion. Attempts at prophylaxis with large doses of atropine usually do no more than make the sputum so viscid that expectoration is even more difficult.

Myasthenic syndrome complicating carcinoma of the bronchus

A myopathy with many features resembling myasthenia gravis was reported in association with malignant disease in the early 1950s. The term 'Eaton–Lambert' syndrome has been applied since, after the authors who described the electromyographic features in 1957. The condition is usually associated with small-cell carcinoma of the bronchus but does occur with other neoplasms and in some instances with no evidence of malignancy. There is now evidence of an autoimmune basis for the myasthenic syndrome with the discovery of antibodies to cationic calcium channels at the motor nerve terminal, as distinct from the antibodies to acetylcholine receptors found at the neuromuscular junction in myasthenia gravis.

The myasthenic syndrome differs from myasthenia gravis in a number of ways (see Table 10.1). It is more common in men, generally in the older age group. Weakness and fatigability of limb muscles, particularly the legs, are the usual presenting features and muscle pains are common. The tendon reflexes are often reduced or absent, and the response to anticholinesterase treatment is poor. Patients with the myasthenic syndrome sometimes notice a transitory increase in strength on activity before fatigue supervenes, whereas those with myasthenia gravis show only progressive fatigue. There are differences too in the responses to muscle relaxants and in electromyographic features. Some patients with the myasthenic syndrome improve considerably if the primary tumour is removed and so they present from time to time for thoracotomy. The majority of patients with small-cell carcinoma of the lung are, however, inoperable at presentation because of distant metastases. In general, they should be managed in the same way as those with myasthenia gravis; every effort should be made to avoid using any muscle relaxant because all the voluntary muscles are vulnerable, not just those in which weakness is symptomatic. Occasional patients with this syndrome will be undiagnosed when they require a diagnostic procedure such as bronchoscopy or mediastinoscopy. If a conventional dose of a muscle relaxant is given inadvertently, postoperative mechanical ventilation until the effect has worn off remains a sensible approach to management. Heroic doses of anticholinesterases are likely to do far more harm than good. Recently, however, there has been increasing interest in the use of aminopyridines in this condition. These drugs increase the release of acetylcholine at the neuromuscular junction, and 3,4-diaminopyridine in particular is used orally to treat the myasthenic syndrome. 3,4-diaminopyridine may also enhance the effects of anticholinesterases in patients with the syndrome inadvertently given a non-depolarizing muscle relaxant.

LUNG TRANSPLANTATION

The first clinically successful heart–lung transplant was carried out in Stanford in 1981. In the ensuing 11 years single-lung, double-lung and bilateral single-lung transplantation have been developed in a number of centres worldwide, following on from the initial success achieved with single-lung transplantation by the Toronto group. Improvements in surgical technique, using an omental wrap around bronchial anastomoses, and the introduction of cyclosporin A as an immunosuppressant (thereby decreasing reliance on corticosteroid therapy) have virtually eliminated problems of bronchial dehiscence with this type of procedure.

Single-lung transplantation is indicated in patients with restrictive lung disease (mainly fibrosing alveolitis) and also in those with obstructive lung disease (principally emphysema). Pulmonary vascular disease, in the absence of congenital heart disease, remains a more controversial indication for single-lung transplantation. Although single-lung transplantation is economic in terms of donor organ usage it is specifically contraindicated in patients with infective lung disease, including those with cystic fibrosis, bronchiectasis and fungal infection. Patients with end-stage cystic fibrosis were initially treated by heart-lung transplantation but more recently *en bloc* double-lung and bilateral single-lung transplantation has been carried out in order to preserve the recipient's own innervated heart and possibly avoid transplant-accelerated coronary artery disease.

In this text on anaesthesia for thoracic surgery the anaesthetic management of single-lung transplantation is described. Aspects of double-lung transplantation are briefly discussed but the reader is referred to texts on cardiac anaesthesia for a full description of anaesthesia for heart-lung transplantation.

Single-lung transplantation

Selection of recipients

The main indications for single-lung transplantation, as stated above, are restrictive and obstructive lung disease in the absence of infection. In both these forms of lung disease one transplanted lung is likely to provide a significant improvement in symptoms and quality of life. In restrictive lung disease the transplanted lung is preferentially ventilated and perfused, and earlier fears that the native lung would overexpand and compress the transplanted lung in obstructive lung disease have largely been unfounded. Transplantation is considered in patients with an estimated life expectancy of 12 to 18 months, although this is notoriously difficult to judge. Lung function is obviously considerably reduced in patients accepted for lung transplantation with a mean forced expired volume in 1 second (FEV_1) of 30% of predicted values and a mean forced vital capacity (FVC) of 35% of predicted values in patients with pulmonary fibrosis in the Newcastle series (Corris, 1991). The age of patients accepted for lung transplantation differs from unit to unit and is, unfortunately, related to donor availability. Patients requiring active respiratory support do not fare well following transplantation and therefore surgical intervention should be planned well before this stage is reached.

Apart from the specific problems of infection and lung function, systemic disease, major organ dysfunction, previous surgery, corticosteroid therapy and cardiac disease may all be contraindications to single-lung transplanta-tion. In relation to concomitant systemic disease, adequate renal and hepatic function are essential, particularly in view of cyclosporin toxicity. Previous thoracic surgery is a relative contraindication to lung transplantation but previous pleurectomy is considered an absolute contraindication in some centres, because of the increased likelihood of perioperative bleeding. Tracheal and bronchial dehiscence are linked to high-dose preoperative steroid therapy. Patients are now accepted for lung transplantation if they are on steroids up to a maximum dose of 7.5 mg of prednisolone daily, provided there is no evidence of steroid-induced thinning of the skin, osteoporosis or myopathy.

Cardiac function is assessed prior to single-lung transplantation and recipients should have adequate ventricular function with no significant coronary artery disease, as assessed echocardiographically and by angio-graphy. Of particular concern is right ventricular function. Many potential recipients will have pulmonary hypertension secondary to their underlying lung disease and it is important that they have sufficient reserve of right ventricular function to withstand the intraoperative period when the pul-monary artery is clamped on the side of surgery and the whole of the cardiac output is directed to the remaining abnormal lung. 'Adequate ventricular function' is difficult to define in the context of single-lung transplantation. Right ventricular ejection fractions as low as 20–30% are considered to be adequate in some centres, particularly as cardiopulmonary bypass can be used intraoperatively in those patients otherwise unable to withstand one-lung anaesthesia and pulmonary artery clamping. Postoperatively, pul-monary vascular resistance, pulmonary artery pressure and right ventricular function are likely to return to normal values in those patients transplanted for pulmonary fibrosis. In this disease the majority of pulmonary blood flow will pass through the relatively normal vascular bed of the transplanted lung leading to a reduction in pulmonary artery pressure postoperatively. In patients with primary pulmonary hypertension or thromboembolic hyper-tension, right ventricular function may not revert to normal postoperatively and this area of surgery remains experimental as far as single-lung trans-plantation is concerned. In these patients, and those with pulmonary hypertension as a result of congenital heart disease, heart-lung transplan-tation remains a therapeutic option.

Donor organs

Donor lungs should be of a suitable size with blood group compatibility to the recipient. Suitable donors are young patients (less than 40 years of age) diagnosed as 'brain dead' who are haemodynamically stable, have had a short period of ventilatory support, no direct pulmonary damage or barotrauma and no previous history of lung disease. Ideally, intended donors should have a relatively normal compliance with adequate gas exchange on 30–35% inspired oxygen concentration and no evidence of frank pulmonary infection. A worldwide shortage of organs for transplantation has led to relaxation of donor criteria in some centres, however, so that the above criteria may now be considered too rigid by some.

Two methods of donor lung preservation are currently in use to allow distant procurement of the organs. One method of preservation entails a hypothermic flush, following pretreatment with a prostacyclin infusion, directly into the pulmonary artery. The constituents of this flush vary from unit to unit but cold donor blood with the addition of anticoagulants, buffer and protein solution is used by the Papworth (UK) group. Mannitol is also added to the solution to reduce interstitial oedema and possibly inhibit complement activity. An alternative approach to organ preservation, used by the Harefield (UK) group, is that of cooling the donor on cardiopulmonary bypass prior to the excision of lungs or a heart-lung block.

Operative technique

Single-lung transplantation can be carried out on the left and the right. The operation is technically easier on the left and a larger lung can be tolerated on this side because of the greater mobility of the diaphragm. If an omental wrap is to be used to 'protect' the bronchial anastomosis a small midline laparotomy is made, with the patient in a supine position, and the omentum mobilized, along with its vascular pedicle, and passed through the diaphragm into the chest. Following closure of the abdomen the patient is placed in a lateral thoracotomy position. A groin is then exposed, and prepared, so that femoral vein to femoral artery cardiopulmonary bypass can be established if necessary.

A standard posterolateral thoracotomy is performed and the proximal pulmonary artery and two pulmonary veins located. The pulmonary artery is temporarily occluded for approximately 5 minutes and if this is well tolerated excision of the diseased lung proceeds. If there is severe hypotension, unacceptable arterial desaturation or a marked rise in contralateral pulmonary artery pressure (see below, p. 243) partial cardiopulmonary bypass is instituted via the femoral vessels.

The donor lung is positioned in the chest following excision of the diseased lung. The pulmonary veins of the donor lung, on their atrial pedicle, are first anastomosed to the recipient left atrium. The pulmonary artery and bronchial anastomoses are then constructed in an end-to-end fashion. The sequence of these anastomoses differs from centre to centre, however, and this may have some bearing on the conduct of anaesthesia (see below, p. 244). Finally, the omental pedicle is wrapped around the bronchial anastomosis. An alternative, and more logical, procedure, also designed to improve bronchial healing may be undertaken. This latter procedure involves anastomosis of the recipient's internal mammary artery to bronchial arteries taken with the donor aorta, thus directly improving bronchial blood flow at the site of anastomosis.

A temporary increase in 'true' shunt (blood flow but no ventilation) is created if the pulmonary blood flow to the donor organ is restored before the bronchial anastomosis is completed. This is rarely a problem, but can be avoided if the vascular clamps are left in place until ventilation of the donor lung is possible. The bronchial anastomosis is constructed first by some surgeons, entirely eliminating the problem.

If cardiopulmonary bypass has been used it is discontinued, in the usual way, once the donor lung has been implanted. Following haemostasis and chest closure the patient is transferred to the intensive care unit. Intermittent positive pressure ventilation is continued via an endotracheal tube.

Anaesthetic technique

Premedication. Little or no premedication is necessary in this group of motivated patients who may be hypoxic and possibly on continuous oxygen therapy. Cyclosporin may be started orally 1–2 hours prior to surgery and azathioprine given intravenously 1 hour prior to surgery or, alternatively, just before the induction of anaesthesia.

Induction and maintenance of anaesthesia. Anaesthesia is induced once intravenous and arterial lines have been inserted percutaneously under local anaesthetic and all monitoring has been established (see Chapter 5). Gross changes in haemodynamic and respiratory status should be avoided where possible by careful technique and appropriate choice of drug therapy. Conacher and colleagues have written extensively on the subject of anaesthesia for single-lung transplantation and recommend the use of etomidate for induction combined with a synthetic opioid such as alfentanil or fentanyl. Vecuronium is a suitable muscle relaxant being largely devoid of histamine-releasing properties. Prophylactic antibiotics are given intravenously during induction of anaesthesia prior to the insertion of venous lines and urethral catheterization.

Anaesthesia can be maintained with fentanyl and a suitable volatile agent such as isoflurane. There is no evidence that volatile agents significantly impair arterial oxygenation during one-lung ventilation for routine thoracic surgery (see Chapter 4) and they have been used satisfactorily during lung transplantation. Nitrous oxide may increase pulmonary vascular resistance and therefore it is prudent to use an inspired gas mixture of air/oxygen.

Monitoring. Comprehensive monitoring should be established as described in Chapter 5. Central venous lines can be inserted in the internal jugular vein on the side of surgery but, as patients will be immunosuppressed in the postoperative period, it is essential to use a sterile technique. Pulse oximetry and end-tidal carbon dioxide analysis are obviously extremely useful during lung transplantation and many, but not all, centres elect to place a pulmonary artery catheter in the pulmonary artery of the lung opposite surgery or in the main pulmonary artery. A pulmonary artery catheter is particularly useful for measuring the effect of unilateral pulmonary artery occlusion on contralateral pulmonary artery pressure and also for monitoring the effect of pulmonary vasodilator drugs at this stage of surgery.

Endobronchial intubation. In the UK a suitable size of sterile double-lumen endobronchial tube is placed in the main bronchus opposite the side of transplantation. This approach is also used in the US but some centres place a double-lumen tube in the left main bronchus, even if left lung transplantation is planned, and others use the Univent tube, an endotracheal tube combined with a bronchial blocker, to provide one-lung anaesthesia. Fibre-optic bronchoscopy is used increasingly to check the position of tubes inserted prior to lung transplantation.

Intraoperative management

Dopamine is prepared and infused at a renal dose, or above, throughout surgery. Mannitol is given intravenously if urine output is inadequate, but excessive fluid loads are avoided. A full range of inotropic and vasodilator drugs (including adrenalin, calcium chloride, aminophylline, isoprenaline, nitroglycerine and sodium nitroprusside) is prepared in bolus and infusion form for use during surgery. These drugs are particularly indicated for the treatment of pulmonary hypertension and right ventricular failure when the pulmonary artery is cross-clamped. The effect of pulmonary vasodilators during this period is often poor, however. If pulmonary hypertension during the cross-clamp period is overwhelming, with near-systemic pulmonary artery pressure, cardiopulmonary bypass is instituted.

Ventilation is continued to both lungs for as long as feasible with an inspired oxygen concentration sufficient to provide adequate oxygen saturation. Some patients will require 100% oxygen to maintain arterial oxygen saturation above 80% during two-lung ventilation and most will require an inspired oxygen concentration of 100% during one-lung ventilation. Arterial carbon dioxide levels are frequently well above normal values, or even the patient's own preoperative values, during two-lung ventilation despite increases in minute ventilation. These levels remain elevated during one-lung ventilation. In patients with obstructive lung disease airtrapping can easily occur during ventilation and if not recognized may result in a significant increase in intrathoracic pressure leading to a decrease in venous return and a fall in cardiac output. A ventilatory pattern with a long expiratory phase may improve the situation but in some instances it is necessary to disconnect the endobronchial tube from the ventilator circuit intermittently and allow passive expiration to atmosphere.

As the pulmonary artery clamp is removed, 1 g of methylprednisolone is given intravenously as part of the immunosuppression regime. As previously discussed unacceptable hypoxaemia can occur at this stage if the bronchial anastomosis has not been completed because the donor lung cannot be ventilated. Various measures have been used to circumvent this problem including separate ventilation of the donor lung via a sterile catheter or ventilator circuit and re-clamping of the pulmonary artery. There is now a tendency to complete the bronchial anastomosis before releasing the pulmonary artery and pulmonary venous clamps so that ventilation of the transplanted lung can begin almost immediately, and as previously stated some surgeons fashion the bronchial anastomosis first.

As two-lung ventilation is commenced, with the donor lung in place, arterial oxygenation and carbon dioxide elimination gradually improve. The inspired oxygen concentration is then slowly decreased to lessen the extent of re-absorption atelectasis and the possibility of hyperoxic damage to the donor lung.

At the end of surgery the endobronchial tube is exchanged for a sterile endotracheal tube. Postoperative ventilation is continued in the intensive care unit.

Postoperative management

The majority of patients are allowed to breathe spontaneously within 36 hours of surgery and are subsequently extubated. Fluid intake is initially restricted and urine output promoted with diuretics and dopamine to avoid accumulation of fluid in the transplanted lung, which is devoid of a functional lymphatic system. Pulmonary oedema in the transplanted lung is the major problem of the first three postoperative days. Antibiotics are continued prophylactically in the early postoperative period and subsequently administered on the basis of sputum cultures.

Immunosuppression regimes vary from unit to unit but azathioprine, antihuman thymocyte globulin and methylprednisolone are commonly given in the immediate postoperative period. Cyclosporin is gradually introduced in the early postoperative period and combined with azathioprine for long-term immunosuppression.

Changes in the donor lung are monitored carefully by daily chest X-rays, serial arterial blood gas analysis and regular spirometry. It may, however, be extremely difficult to differentiate between graft rejection and an opportunistic lung infection. The symptoms of cough, dyspnoea and chest tightness are similar in both conditions as are the physical signs, of crepitations and wheeze, on auscultation. The chest X-ray may also be unhelpful with bilateral pulmonary shadows evident in both conditions. Changes in simple lung function tests of FEV_1 and FVC can be relatively sensitive for rejection, particularly in the later postoperative period. A significant decrease in values for FEV_1 and FVC over two consecutive days warrants further investigation. If rejection or an opportunistic lung infection is suspected transbronchial lung biopsy and lung lavage are undertaken to define the problem. Appropriate therapy can then be started. Common opportunistic pathogens include cytomegalovirus, *Pneumocystis carinii* and herpes simplex virus. Aspergillus infection may, additionally, be superimposed on those patients with a pre-existing cytomegalovirus pneumonia.

Obliterative bronchiolitis remains a major long-term complication of both heart-lung and single-lung transplantation. This process is defined as irreversible severe airflow obstruction, where the decline in lung function has not been arrested by the use of augmented immunosuppression (Dennis & Higenbottam, 1991). Histologically there is obliteration of the bronchioli which are left as fibrous bands extending out to the pleura, with associated dilatation and bronchiectasis of the proximal airways. Obliterative bronchiolitis has an incidence of up to 20–40% in single-lung recipients and commonly occurs between 3 months to 2 years after transplantation. The aetiology of the condition remains obscure but is thought to be a result of chronic rejection and/or donor organ ischaemia. Close monitoring of lung function, allowing early treatment of rejection episodes, appears to reduce the incidence of obliterative bronchiolitis in single-lung recipients.

Double-lung and bilateral single-lung transplantation

En bloc double-lung transplantation, via a mediansternotomy, was developed for use in patients with respiratory disease yet good myocardial function. Patients with bilateral lung sepsis, such as cystic fibrosis, are suitable candidates for this procedure but initial problems with tracheal dehiscence has led to the development of sequential bilateral single-lung transplantation as an alternative procedure. This latter operation is carried out via a transverse bilateral thoracotomy with horizontal division of the sternum.

Double-lung transplantation is carried out using cardiopulmonary bypass. Full heparinization is required so that postoperative bleeding is a major problem, as it is following the use of cardiopulmonary bypass for single-lung transplantation. Intraoperative ventilation can be managed with a short endotracheal tube.

Bilateral single-lung transplantation can be accomplished without the use of cardiopulmonary bypass, in many cases, but intraoperative ventilation is more problematical. A left-sided double-lumen endobronchial tube, the Univent endotracheal tube/blocker combination (see Chapter 5), and a standard endotracheal tube combined with a Fogarty catheter as a bronchial blocker have all been used to provide satisfactory ventilation during bilateral single-lung transplantation.

FURTHER READING

Bronchopulmonary lavage

Cohen E. & Eisenkraft J.B. (1990) Bronchopulmonary lavage: effects on oxygenation and haemodynamics. *Journal of Cardiothoracic Anesthesia*, **4**, 119–130.
Costello J.F., Moriarty D.C. & Branthwaite M.A. (1975) Diagnosis and management of alveolar proteinosis: the role of electron microscopy. *Thorax*, **30**, 121–132.
Lippman M., Mok M.S. & Wasserman K. (1977) Anaesthetic management for children with alveolar proteinosis using extracorporeal circulation. *British Journal of Anaesthesia*, **49**, 173–175.
McKenzie B., Wood R.E. & Bailey A. (1989) Airway management for unilateral lung lavage in children. *Anesthesiology*, **70**, 550–554.
Spragg R.G., Benumof J.L. & Alfery D.D. (1982) New methods for the performance of unilateral lung lavage. *Anesthesiology*, **57**, 535–542.

Mediastinal tumours

Akhtar T.M., Ridley S. & Best C.J. (1991) Unusual presentation of acute upper airway obstruction caused by an anterior mediastinal mass. *British Journal of Anaesthesia*, **67**, 632–634.
Bray R.J. & Fernandes F.J. (1982) Mediastinal tumour causing airway obstruction in anaesthetised children. *Anaesthesia*, **37**, 571–575.

Brown K., Aberle D.R., Batra P. & Steckel R.J. (1990) Current use of imaging in the evaluation of primary mediastinal masses. *Chest*, **2**, 466–473.

Ferrari L.R. & Bedford R.F. (1990) General anesthesia prior to treatment of mediastinal masses in pediatric cancer patients. *Anesthesiology*, **72**, 991–995.

Fletcher R. & Nordstrom L. (1986) The effects of gas exchange of a large mediastinal tumour. *Anaesthesia*, **41**, 1135–1138.

Gothard J.W.W. (1989) Anaesthesia for thoracic malignancy. In: Filshie J. & Robbie D.S. (eds) *Anaesthesia and Malignant Disease*. Edward Arnold, London.

Hall D.K. & Friedman M. (1975) Extracorporeal oxygenation for induction of anesthesia in a patient with an intrathoracic tumour. *Anesthesiology*, **42**, 493–495.

John R.E. & Narang V.P.S. (1988) A boy with an anterior mediastinal mass. *Anaesthesia*, **43**, 864–866.

Klein D.S. & Wilds P.R. (1983) Pulmonary toxicity of antineoplastic agents: anesthetic and post-operative implications. *Canadian Anaesthetists Society Journal*, **30**, 399–405.

Mackie A.M. & Watson C.B. (1984) Anaesthesia and mediastinal masses. *Anaesthesia*, **39**, 899–903.

Neuman G.G., Weingarten A.E., Abramovitz R.M., Kushins L.G., Abramson A.L. & Ladner W. (1984) The anesthetic management of the patient with an anterior mediastinal mass. *Anesthesiology*, **60**, 144–147.

Schwartz A.J. & Howie (1987) Case conference — mediastinal mass in a 57-year-old man. *Journal of Cardiothoracic Anesthesia*, **1**, 71–79.

Younker D., Clark R. & Coveler L. (1989) Fibreoptic endobronchial intubation for resection of an anterior mediastinal mass. *Anesthesiology*, **70**, 144–146.

Myasthenia gravis and myasthenic syndrome

Eaton L.M. & Lambert E.H. (1957) Electromyography and electrical stimulation of nerves in disease with motor units. Observations on myasthenic syndrome associated with malignant tumours. *Journal of the American Medical Association*, **163**, 1117–1124.

Eisenkraft J.B. (1987) Myasthenia gravis and thymic surgery — anaesthetic considerations. In: Gothard J.W.W. (ed.) *Thoracic Anaesthesia. Clinical Anaesthesiology*, Vol. 1, pp. 133–162. Baillière Tindall, London.

Nilsson E. & Meretoja O.A. (1990) Vecuronium dose-response and maintenance requirements in patients with myasthenia gravis. *Anesthesiology*, **73**, 28–32.

Sakura S., Saito Y., Maeda M. & Kosaka Y. (1991) Epidural analgesia in Eaton–Lambert myasthenic syndrome. *Anaesthesia*, **46**, 560–562.

Small S., Hassan H.A., Lennon V.A., Brown R.H., Carr D.B. & Armendi A.D. (1992) Anesthesia for an unsuspected Lambert–Eaton myasthenic syndrome with autoantibodies and occult small cell lung carcinoma. *Anesthesiology*, **76**, 142–145.

Telford R.J. & Hollway T.E. (1990) The myasthenic syndrome: anaesthesia in a patient treated with 3-4, diaminopyridine. *British Journal of Anaesthesia*, **64**, 363–366.

Lung transplantation

Bradley J.T. & Lawrence C.S. (1991) Anesthetic and postoperative management of single-lung transplantation. *Journal of Cardiothoracic and Vascular Anesthesia*, **5**, 266–267.

Cooper J.D., Patterson G.A., Grossman R. & Maurer J. & The Toronto Lung Transplantation Group (1989) Double-lung transplant for advanced chronic obstructive lung disease. *American Review of Respiratory Diseases*, **139**, 303–307.

Conacher I.D. (1988) Isolated lung transplantation: a review of problems and guide to anaesthesia. *British Journal of Anaesthesia*, **61**, 468–474.

Conacher I.D., McNally B., Choudry A.K. & McGregor C.G.A. (1988) Anaesthesia for isolated lung transplantation. *British Journal of Anaesthesia*, **60**, 588–591.

Conacher I.D., Dark J., Hilton C.J. & Corris P. (1990) Isolated lung transplantation for pulmonary fibrosis. *Anaesthesia*, **45**, 971–975.

Corris P.A. (1991) Patient selection and preoperative work-up. In: Mitchell D.M. (ed.) *Recent Advances in Respiratory Medicine*, Vol. 5, pp. 251–257. Mini symposium on lung transplantation. Churchill Livingstone, Edinburgh.

Dark J. & Cooper J.D. (1987) Transplantation of the lungs. *British Journal of Hospital Medicine*, **37**, 443–445.

Dennis C. & Higenbottam T.W. (1991) Postoperative complication and follow-up. In: Mitchell D.M. (ed.) *Recent Advances in Respiratory Medicine*, Vol. 5, pp. 279–289. Mini symposium on lung transplantation. Churchill Livingstone, Edinburgh.

Editorial (1992) Lung transplantation. *Lancet*, **339**, 1021–1022.

Gayes J.M., Giron L., Nissen M.D. & Plut D. (1990) Anesthetic considerations for patients undergoing double-lung transplantation. *Journal of Cardiothoracic Anesthesia*, **4**, 486–498.

Lee B.S., Sarnquist F.H. & Starnes V.A. (1992) Anesthesia for bilateral single-lung transplantation. *Journal of Cardiothoracic and Vascular Anesthesia*, **6**, 201–203.

Robertson K.M. & Cook D.R. (1990) Perioperative management of the multiorgan donor. *Anesthesia and Analgesia*, **70**, 546–556.

Scheller M.S., Kriet J.M., Smith C.M. & Jamieson S.W. (1992) Airway management during anesthesia for double-lung transplantation using a single-lumen endotracheal tube with an enclosed bronchial blocker. *Journal of Cardiothoracic and Vascular Anesthesia*, **6**, 204–207.

The Toronto Lung Transplant Group (1988) Experience with single-lung transplantation for pulmonary fibrosis. *Journal of the American Medical Association*, **259**, 2258–2262.

Index

Note: Page numbers in *Italics* refer to figures and/or tables